# Vagus Nerve Exercises

Your Guide to Activate and Stimulate the Vagus Nerve to Release Stress and Ignite Mental Clarit

*Harper Ripmar*

# Table of Contents

# Introduction

# Welcome to a Journey of Healing and Clarity

## Your first step towards unlocking mental clarity and stress relief

Welcome to the first steps on your journey to unlocking mental clarity and stress relief. This chapter is more than just an introduction; it's an invitation to a transformative experience that will resonate deeply with your current lifestyle and aspirations.

Imagine a typical day in your life. You're likely juggling numerous responsibilities: a demanding career, family obligations, and the pursuit of personal interests, all within the bustling environment of an urban area. Amidst this whirlwind of activity, you find solace in your hobbies - yoga, meditation, and reading. They are not just pastimes; they are your sanctuaries of peace and personal growth. This book aims to enhance these moments of tranquility, offering you tools to elevate your mental clarity and alleviate stress.

Your interest in wellness is evident. You follow influencers who advocate for a balanced lifestyle, listen to podcasts that delve into the mind-body connection, and are always on the lookout for ways to enrich your wellbeing. This shows a deep commitment to not just understanding but truly embodying a lifestyle that prioritizes mental and physical health.

The journey towards unlocking mental clarity and stress relief starts with understanding that the solution lies within you. The Vagus Nerve, a key focus of this book, is your internal pathway to tranquility and clarity. This nerve, wandering from the brainstem down to your abdomen, touches almost every organ and is pivotal in regulating stress responses. By learning to stimulate and activate this nerve, you can directly influence your mental state, turning the key to unlock a calmer, more focused version of yourself.

Stress, an all-too-familiar companion in modern life, often seems like an insurmountable challenge. It creeps into your life, uninvited, and can overshadow your days with anxiety and unrest. However, with the right approach, stress can be managed and even transformed into a positive force. This book will guide you through simple yet effective exercises that you can incorporate into your daily routine, exercises that are specially designed to engage and stimulate the Vagus Nerve, thereby reducing stress and enhancing mental clarity.

Consider the power of breathing, an act so simple yet so profound. Breathing techniques are among the first and most accessible tools to stimulate the Vagus Nerve. Through controlled and mindful breathing, you can send signals of calm to your body, mitigating the fight-or-flight response that stress induces. These techniques are not just theoretical; they are practical, backed by science, and can be seamlessly integrated into your everyday life.

In your pursuit of wellness, you have probably experienced the benefits of yoga and meditation. These practices are not just physical exercises; they are gateways to understanding and harmonizing your body and mind. This book will delve into how these practices specifically activate the Vagus Nerve, enhancing their effectiveness in your journey towards mental clarity and stress relief.

Your quest for balance and clarity is not just a personal journey; it's a journey that resonates with your role in your family and community. The skills and knowledge you acquire will not only transform your life but also positively influence those around you. As you learn to manage stress and nurture mental clarity, you become a beacon of calm and focus, inspiring and supporting your loved ones in their own journeys.

While your busy lifestyle might make it seem challenging to incorporate new practices, this book is designed to offer strategies that fit seamlessly into your schedule. Whether it's a breathing exercise during a short break at work or a mindfulness practice before bed, you will find ways to make these exercises a natural part of your day.

As you turn the pages of this book, remember that each chapter is a step forward in your journey. A journey that doesn't require drastic changes but rather, embraces small, consistent practices that build over time. You are not just reading a book; you are embarking on a path of transformation. A transformation that promises to bring more clarity, more peace, and a stronger sense of control over your life's stresses.

In conclusion, your journey towards mental clarity and stress relief begins with an understanding of the power that lies within you - the power of the Vagus Nerve. By learning to activate and stimulate this nerve, you unlock the door to a calmer, more focused state of mind. This book is your guide, your companion in this journey, offering practical, science-backed strategies that are tailored to fit into your lifestyle. Welcome to the first step of a transformative journey, a journey towards healing, clarity, and a balanced life.

# How this book will transform your life

Transformation – a word often promised, yet seldom delivered in its truest sense. "How this book will transform your life" is not just a chapter title; it's a commitment, a journey we embark on together through the pages of this book. You, a discerning individual in your prime, living a life filled with responsibilities and ambitions, are about to unlock a powerful tool for personal growth and well-being.

Imagine waking up each morning with a newfound clarity, a sense of calm that carries you through the hustle of urban life. This isn't just a dream; it's a tangible reality that this book aims to facilitate. As someone who cherishes yoga, meditation, and a continuous quest for knowledge, you have already laid the groundwork for this transformation. What this book offers is a deep dive into understanding and harnessing the power of the Vagus Nerve – a key player in your mental and physical wellness.

The Vagus Nerve, often overlooked, is your internal dial for controlling stress and anxiety. By learning to stimulate this nerve, you will be taking control of your body's relaxation response, shifting the balance from a state of constant alertness to one of calm and focus. This shift is not just about feeling relaxed; it's about enhancing your cognitive abilities, improving your decision-making, and nurturing a sense of well-being that permeates all aspects of life.

Your weekends spent in parks, your commitment to wellness retreats, and your avid consumption of wellness media, all reflect a deep desire for a balanced, healthy lifestyle. This book aligns perfectly with these pursuits. Each chapter is crafted not only to educate but to provide practical, actionable strategies that can be incorporated into your busy schedule. From breathing exercises that can be practiced during a short break at work, to physical exercises that align with your yoga routine, every aspect is designed to fit seamlessly into your life.

Moreover, the transformation promised in this book goes beyond individual benefits. It extends to your interactions with family, friends, and colleagues. As you practice the exercises and integrate the teachings, you will find yourself becoming a source of calm and strength to those around you. Your improved mental clarity and reduced stress levels will not only enhance your personal well-being but also positively influence your relationships and professional life.

Furthermore, this book acknowledges your preference for visual and interactive content. Expect to find engaging illustrations, easy-to-follow guides, and links to supplementary digital content that will enrich your learning experience. This multimodal approach ensures that the concepts and exercises are not only understood but also retained and applied.

Transformation is also about overcoming challenges, and this book doesn't shy away from addressing the complexities of stress and mental health in modern life. It doesn't offer oversimplified solutions or magical cures. Instead, it provides a nuanced, in-depth understanding of how the Vagus Nerve interacts with your body and mind, backed by scientific research and real-life case studies. This approach ensures that the transformation you experience is grounded in reality, sustainable, and deeply rooted in scientific understanding.

As you delve into the pages of this book, expect to embark on a journey that is as enlightening as it is empowering. You will learn not just about the Vagus Nerve but also about yourself – your body's responses to stress, your mental triggers, and your untapped potential for resilience and clarity. The transformation promised here is not just about reducing anxiety or stress; it's about redefining your relationship with your own mind and body.

In conclusion, this book is more than just a collection of exercises and theories. It's a pathway to a transformed life – a life where stress and anxiety are managed effectively, where mental clarity is the norm, and where your well-being is prioritized. It's a commitment to not just learn, but to apply, to not just read, but to experience. As you turn each page, remember that every word is a step towards a more balanced, focused, and fulfilling life. Welcome to a transformation that begins with knowledge and culminates in a profound understanding and mastery of your own well-being.

# Part I: Understanding the Vagus Nerve

# Chapter 1: The Vagus Nerve Unveiled

## Anatomy and functions

The Vagus Nerve, often termed as the 'wandering nerve', is a marvel of human anatomy, a testament to the intricate and intelligent design of our bodies. In this chapter, 'Anatomy and Functions', we will explore the vast and varied landscape of this remarkable nerve, understanding its structure, its myriad functions, and its crucial role in maintaining our physical and mental well-being.

Embarking on this exploration, it's important to first understand the basic anatomy of the Vagus Nerve. This nerve is the longest of the cranial nerves, extending from the brainstem through the neck and down into the chest and abdomen. It's a bi-directional highway, conveying sensory information from the body to the brain and motor control signals from the brain to the body. But to merely call it a nerve does not do justice to its vast network and influence. It touches almost every organ in the body, from the throat to the heart, the lungs to the digestive system.

The functions of the Vagus Nerve are as diverse as its path through the body. It's like a master conductor, orchestrating a symphony of critical bodily functions. One of its key roles is in regulating the autonomic nervous system, which controls our involuntary bodily functions. This includes managing heart rate, controlling muscle movement, overseeing digestive processes, and regulating respiratory rate. It acts as a mediator between the mind and body, translating physical sensations into emotional responses and vice versa.

In the realm of heart health, the Vagus Nerve plays a pivotal role in controlling heart rate and blood pressure. It sends signals to slow the heart rate, promoting calm and relaxation. This function is particularly significant in today's fast-paced world, where stress and anxiety are rampant. By learning to stimulate the Vagus Nerve, individuals can effectively manage their heart rate, reducing the risk of heart-related issues.

The nerve's influence extends to the lungs as well. It helps regulate breathing patterns, which is why breathing exercises are often recommended for stimulating the Vagus Nerve. Such exercises not only improve lung function but also trigger relaxation responses in the body, promoting a state of calm and reducing stress levels.

In the digestive system, the Vagus Nerve is essential for controlling muscle movements that propel food through the gastrointestinal tract. It also affects the release of digestive enzymes, playing a crucial role in the digestion and absorption of nutrients. This highlights the importance of gut health in overall well-being and the interconnectedness of the body's various systems.

Moreover, the Vagus Nerve is a key player in the body's inflammation response. It helps regulate immune system activity, reducing inflammation levels in the body. This is crucial, as chronic inflammation is linked to numerous health conditions, including heart disease, diabetes, and arthritis.

But perhaps the most fascinating aspect of the Vagus Nerve is its role in the mind-body connection. It's a primary component of the parasympathetic nervous system, often referred to as the 'rest and digest' system. This system counteracts the stress responses triggered by the sympathetic nervous system. By stimulating the Vagus Nerve, individuals can actively shift their body's response from stress to relaxation, promoting mental clarity and reducing anxiety.

In mental health, the Vagus Nerve influences mood and stress levels. It's involved in transmitting neurotransmitters like acetylcholine and norepinephrine, which play a significant role in mood regulation. This has implications for treating conditions like depression and anxiety, offering a natural pathway to manage these conditions through Vagus Nerve stimulation.

As we delve deeper into the anatomy and functions of the Vagus Nerve, we begin to understand its profound impact on our overall health. It's not just a nerve; it's a critical component of our body's communication network, a key to unlocking better health and well-being. By learning to stimulate and regulate this nerve, we can tap into its vast potential, improving our physical and mental health in myriad ways.

The Vagus Nerve is a bridge between mind and body, an essential tool in our quest for health and wellness. Its extensive reach and diverse functions make it a key focus in holistic health approaches. As we move forward in this book, we will explore practical ways to stimulate and harness the power of the Vagus

Nerve, unlocking its potential to transform our health and enrich our lives.

## Its role in the mind-body connection

The role of the Vagus Nerve in the mind-body connection is a fascinating and integral part of understanding holistic health. This connection, often referred to as the mind-body link, is the invisible thread that ties together our physical sensations and our mental states. It's a dance of communication between our thoughts, feelings, and bodily responses, and the Vagus Nerve plays a central role in this intricate ballet.

In the realm of the mind-body connection, the Vagus Nerve acts as a mediator, a bridge that conveys messages between the brain and the body. This nerve, wandering through the body, carries signals that affect our emotional and physiological states. It's a conduit through which our mental state can influence our physical health and vice versa.

Consider for a moment the experience of stress or anxiety. These are not just mental states; they manifest physically. Your heart races, your breathing quickens, your muscles tense. This is the sympathetic nervous system in action, preparing your body for a 'fight or flight' response. However, in our modern world, these responses are often triggered by non-life-threatening stressors, like work pressure or daily commutes. Here, the Vagus Nerve plays a crucial role in counteracting these effects by activating the parasympathetic nervous system, often termed the 'rest and digest' system.

The Vagus Nerve, when stimulated, sends a message to your body to slow down. It lowers the heart rate, relaxes muscles, and regulates breathing. This shift from a state of heightened alertness to one of calm is essential for maintaining balance in our lives. It's not just about feeling relaxed; it's about enabling the body to recover and maintain equilibrium.

This nerve's influence on the mind-body connection extends to various physiological processes that are fundamental to our well-being. In the digestive system, for instance, the Vagus Nerve helps regulate the process of digestion, affecting how we absorb nutrients and maintain gut health. The health of our gut, often called the 'second brain', has been shown to have a significant impact on our mental state, influencing mood and emotional well-being.

In the realm of mental health, the Vagus Nerve's role in regulating neurotransmitters is crucial. It affects the release of chemicals like serotonin and dopamine, which play a vital role in mood regulation. This has profound implications for the treatment of mental health conditions like depression and anxiety. By learning to stimulate the Vagus Nerve, individuals can potentially influence their mental state, finding relief from the symptoms of these conditions.

Moreover, the Vagus Nerve's role in the mind-body connection is not just reactive; it's also proactive. Regular stimulation of this nerve through practices like deep breathing, meditation, and yoga can enhance our resilience to stress. It's like training a muscle; the more we engage this nerve, the stronger our mind-body connection becomes, allowing us to better manage stress and maintain mental clarity.

For you, our reader, who spends weekends exploring parks, attending wellness retreats, and engaging in yoga and meditation, understanding and leveraging the Vagus Nerve's role in the mind-body connection can be transformative. It aligns with your lifestyle and interests, offering a scientifically grounded approach to enhancing your holistic well-being.

In this fast-paced world, where we are constantly bombarded with stimuli, the ability to maintain a balance between our mental and physical states is invaluable. The Vagus Nerve, in its role as a mediator of the mind-body connection, offers a natural pathway to achieving this balance. It's a tool that, when understood and utilized, can elevate our quality of life, enhancing our mental clarity, emotional stability, and overall physical health.

The Vagus Nerve's role in the mind-body connection is a testament to the interconnectedness of our mental and physical health. It's a critical component in understanding how our bodies respond to our mental states and how our mental states can influence our physical well-being. As we continue to explore the wonders of the Vagus Nerve, we uncover more ways to harness its power, opening doors to a healthier, more balanced life.

# Case studies: Real-life impacts of a stimulated vagus nerve

The profound impact of stimulating the Vagus Nerve is best illustrated through real-life case studies. These narratives provide tangible evidence of how this nerve, when engaged effectively, can transform lives. In this section, we delve into several case studies that showcase the real-life impacts of a stimulated Vagus Nerve on individuals who mirror your demographic and share similar interests and lifestyles.

## Case Study 1: The Corporate Executive

John, a 42-year-old corporate executive living in a bustling metropolitan area, faced chronic stress and hypertension, common issues among individuals in high-pressure jobs. His routine was a whirlwind of meetings, business trips, and extended work hours. Despite a successful career and a comfortable lifestyle, John's physical and mental health were declining.

After attending a wellness seminar, John learned about the Vagus Nerve's role in stress management. He began practicing deep breathing exercises and mindfulness meditation, focusing on stimulating his Vagus Nerve. Over several months, John noticed a significant decrease in his stress levels and a remarkable improvement in his blood pressure readings. The simple act of regularly stimulating his Vagus Nerve had a profound impact on his overall health.

## Case Study 2: The Yoga Enthusiast

Sarah, 38, an avid yoga practitioner and reader of wellness literature, struggled with anxiety and digestive issues. Despite her active lifestyle and healthy eating habits, she found herself frequently overwhelmed by anxiety, which adversely affected her digestive health.

Upon learning about the connection between the Vagus Nerve and gut health, Sarah incorporated specific yoga poses known to stimulate the Vagus Nerve into her daily routine. She also adopted guided meditations that focused on deep, diaphragmatic breathing. Over time, Sarah experienced a noticeable improvement in her digestive health and a significant reduction in her anxiety levels. The integration of Vagus Nerve stimulation into her yoga practice proved to be a key factor in her journey to better health.

## Case Study 3: The Dedicated Parent

Michael, a 45-year-old father of two, balanced a demanding job with an active family life. While he enjoyed spending weekends with his family and exploring nature, he often felt fatigued and experienced occasional bouts of depression. Michael's busy lifestyle left him with little time for self-care.

After attending a health conference, Michael learned about the Vagus Nerve's role in mood regulation. He began practicing simple, quick techniques to stimulate his Vagus Nerve, such as humming and gargling, which he could easily incorporate into his daily routine. These activities, coupled with regular walks in nature, led to a noticeable improvement in his mood and energy levels. Michael found that stimulating his Vagus Nerve helped him achieve a more balanced and enjoyable life.

## Case Study 4: The Wellness Advocate

Emma, a 39-year-old wellness blogger, was passionate about mental health and well-being. Despite her knowledge and interest in wellness, she faced challenges with sleep disturbances and chronic neck tension. Emma's commitment to her blog and social media presence, while fulfilling, often led to long hours in front of a computer.

Upon researching the Vagus Nerve, Emma decided to experiment with sound therapy, particularly chanting and singing, to stimulate the nerve. She also incorporated Vagus Nerve massages into her routine. Remarkably, these practices led to improved sleep quality and a reduction in neck tension. Emma's experience highlighted the versatility of Vagus Nerve stimulation techniques and their potential to address a variety of health concerns.

These case studies reflect the diverse ways in which stimulating the Vagus Nerve can positively impact health and well-being. From managing stress and anxiety to improving digestive health and mood regulation, the benefits are wide-ranging. Each individual's story underscores the importance of incorporating simple yet effective Vagus Nerve stimulation techniques into one's daily routine.

For you, our reader, these real-life examples provide not just inspiration but also a practical blueprint for enhancing your own health. Whether through breathing exercises, yoga, mindfulness, or other methods, the potential of the Vagus Nerve to transform your life is immense. As you journey through this book, consider these stories as a testament to the power of the Vagus Nerve and an invitation to explore its benefits in your own life.

# Chapter 2: The Science of Stress and Mental Clarity

## How stress affects your body and mind

Understanding how stress affects your body and mind is crucial in the journey towards mental clarity and well-being. Stress, a common experience in the fast-paced lives of urban dwellers, especially among those in high-income, high-pressure environments, is not just a fleeting emotional state. It has tangible, profound effects on both your physical and mental health.

When you encounter a stressful situation, your body responds in a way that's hardwired into your biology, a legacy of our ancestors' need for survival. This response, often referred to as the 'fight or flight' reaction, involves a series of hormonal and physiological changes. The adrenal glands release stress hormones like cortisol and adrenaline. These hormones increase your heart rate, elevate your blood pressure, and boost energy supplies. While this response is crucial for reacting to immediate threats, chronic activation due to ongoing stress can lead to detrimental health effects.

Physically, chronic stress can manifest in numerous ways. It can contribute to headaches, muscle tension, fatigue, and sleep disturbances. Over time, elevated cortisol levels can lead to more severe health issues like cardiovascular diseases, including hypertension and heart attacks, obesity, and type 2 diabetes. Your digestive system also takes a hit under stress, leading to symptoms like indigestion, heartburn, or exacerbation of existing conditions like irritable bowel syndrome (IBS).

The impact of stress on your mental health is equally significant. It can cloud your thinking, affecting your concentration and decision-making capabilities. This mental fog, a direct result of the stress response, can hamper your productivity and creativity – vital attributes in your professional and personal life. Stress is also closely linked to mental health disorders such as anxiety and depression. It can create a vicious cycle, where stress exacerbates these conditions, which in turn, increase your stress levels.

Moreover, stress can influence your behavior in ways that may further impact your health. Under stress, some people tend to eat more or choose unhealthier foods, use substances like alcohol or tobacco, or withdraw from social connections. These coping mechanisms, while providing short-term relief, can lead to long-term health problems and further compound the stress you experience.

For someone immersed in a lifestyle that includes yoga, meditation, and a focus on wellness, understanding the impact of stress is the first step in mitigating its effects. Practices like yoga and meditation are not just tools for relaxation; they are powerful strategies to counteract the physical and mental effects of stress. They help in regulating the stress response, bringing a sense of calm and clarity to your mind and body.

Stress is a multifaceted challenge that affects both your body and mind. Its effects are far-reaching, influencing your physical health, mental clarity, emotional stability, and overall quality of life. As you continue to explore the science of stress and mental clarity, remember that understanding the enemy – stress – is the first step in mastering it. Armed with this knowledge, you can employ the right tools and strategies, such as the practices detailed in this book, to manage stress effectively and improve your overall well-being.

# The vagus nerve's role in cognitive function

The Vagus Nerve's role in cognitive function is a subject of burgeoning interest, especially in a demographic attuned to the nuances of mental wellness and personal development. As a critical component of the parasympathetic nervous system, the Vagus Nerve not only plays a vital role in regulating stress responses but also significantly influences cognitive functions like attention, memory, and decision-making.

Cognitive function encompasses various mental abilities, including learning, thinking, reasoning, remembering, problem-solving, decision-making, and attention. It's the bedrock upon which we build our daily lives, from simple tasks to complex professional and personal interactions. The Vagus Nerve influences these abilities in several ways.

First, consider the role of the Vagus Nerve in regulating stress. When the body faces stress, the 'fight or flight' response kicks in, and cognitive resources are redirected towards survival instincts. This response, while beneficial in short-term, high-stress situations, can impair cognitive function if prolonged. The Vagus Nerve acts as a counterbalance to this response. By stimulating this nerve, the body shifts towards the 'rest and digest' state, wherein the body and mind are calmer and more conducive to cognitive tasks.

Moreover, the Vagus Nerve affects the brain's neurotransmitter systems, which are crucial for cognitive function. It influences the release of acetylcholine, a neurotransmitter associated with attention and learning. A well-functioning Vagus Nerve ensures optimal levels of acetylcholine, leading to better focus and memory retention. This is particularly relevant for individuals in their 40s, who may begin to experience subtle changes in memory and attention.

The Vagus Nerve also impacts the brain's health directly. It promotes neurogenesis – the creation of new neurons – and supports neural plasticity, which is the brain's ability to change and adapt throughout life. These processes are fundamental for learning and memory. Stimulating the Vagus Nerve, through practices such as deep breathing or yoga, can enhance these brain functions, leading to improved cognitive abilities.

For the audience this book caters to – individuals who are not just career-oriented but also deeply involved in personal growth and wellness – understanding the cognitive benefits of a healthy Vagus Nerve is crucial. Many in this demographic already engage in activities like yoga and meditation, which indirectly stimulate the Vagus Nerve. Recognizing the direct cognitive benefits of these practices can add a new layer of intention and benefit to their routine.

Moreover, the Vagus Nerve's influence on cognition extends to emotional intelligence. Emotional intelligence, a critical component of effective interpersonal communication and self-understanding, benefits from the calming, balancing effects of a well-regulated Vagus Nerve. In an age where emotional intelligence is recognized as a key skill in both personal and professional realms, this aspect of cognitive function cannot be overlooked.

In conclusion, the Vagus Nerve's role in cognitive function is multifaceted and profound. Its influence spans from the biochemical – regulating neurotransmitters, to the physiological – maintaining the balance between stress and relaxation, all of which are critical for optimal cognitive functioning. For an audience committed to maintaining a balanced, introspective, and growth-oriented lifestyle, understanding and harnessing the power of the Vagus Nerve can be a game-changer in enhancing cognitive abilities and overall mental clarity.

# The connection between the vagus nerve and mental health

The connection between the Vagus Nerve and mental health is a topic of paramount importance, especially considering the stressful lifestyle of urban dwellers in the upper-middle-class demographic. This nerve, often overlooked, plays a pivotal role in regulating many aspects of our mental health. Understanding this connection is crucial for anyone seeking holistic approaches to improve their mental well-being.

The Vagus Nerve is like the body's superhighway, transmitting signals between the brain and various organs. It is a core part of the parasympathetic nervous system, often referred to as the "rest and digest" system. This system acts as a counterbalance to the sympathetic nervous system's "fight or flight" response.

In the context of mental health, the Vagus Nerve helps regulate mood and anxiety levels.

When you experience stress, the sympathetic nervous system triggers a flood of stress hormones, preparing the body for a quick response. While this is beneficial for immediate, short-term situations, chronic stress can lead to an overactivation of this response, contributing to anxiety and depression. The Vagus Nerve, through its calming influence, helps dampen this response, promoting a state of relaxation and recovery.

Stimulation of the Vagus Nerve has been shown to increase levels of neurotransmitters such as GABA, which have a calming effect on the brain. This is particularly significant for people dealing with anxiety disorders. By increasing GABA levels, Vagus Nerve stimulation can reduce anxiety symptoms, creating a sense of calmness and improving overall mental health.

Moreover, the Vagus Nerve influences the production and release of other mood-regulating neurotransmitters, including serotonin and dopamine. Imbalances in these neurotransmitters are often linked to depression. Thus, maintaining a healthy Vagus Nerve function is essential for emotional regulation and can be a natural, effective way to manage and prevent depressive symptoms.

This connection is of particular interest to the demographic engaging in yoga and meditation. These practices are known to stimulate the Vagus Nerve, thereby enhancing its ability to regulate mood and stress responses. It's not just about the physical postures or the act of meditation; it's about how these practices activate the Vagus Nerve, leading to improved mental health.

Furthermore, the Vagus Nerve's role in gut-brain communication is another vital aspect of its connection to mental health. The nerve plays a significant role in the functioning of the gut, which has been dubbed the "second brain" due to its vast network of neurons. There is increasing evidence to suggest that gut health significantly impacts mental health, with the Vagus Nerve being a key mediator in this gut-brain axis.

In the end, the Vagus Nerve's connection to mental health is multifaceted and profound. Its role in regulating stress responses, neurotransmitter levels, and gut-brain communication makes it an essential focus for anyone seeking to improve their mental well-being. For individuals who are well-versed in wellness literature and practices, understanding and harnessing the power of the Vagus Nerve can be a transformative step towards achieving mental clarity and emotional balance. As we continue to explore this connection, it becomes clear that the Vagus Nerve is not just a physical entity but a bridge to a healthier, more harmonious state of mind.

# Part II: The Path to Mental Clarity

# Chapter 3: Breathing Techniques for Vagus Nerve Stimulation

## The science of breathing

The science of breathing, often overlooked in its simplicity, is a profound and vital aspect of human physiology, particularly relevant to the well-being of a demographic engaged in the pursuit of balance and wellness. Breathing is not just a basic life function; it's an intricate process that influences our mental, physical, and emotional health. Understanding the science behind it is crucial for anyone looking to harness its power, especially in stimulating the Vagus Nerve for improved health outcomes.

Breathing is an autonomic process, meaning it occurs automatically, but it's unique in that it can be consciously controlled. This characteristic makes it a powerful tool for influencing our body's responses. When we breathe, we inhale oxygen and exhale carbon dioxide, a basic exchange essential for life. However, the manner in which we breathe – the depth, rhythm, and rate – has profound effects on our body's systems.

At the core of the science of breathing is the concept of the mind-body connection. Our breathing patterns are closely linked to our emotional states. When stressed, our breaths tend to be shallow and rapid, triggering the sympathetic nervous system, which is responsible for the 'fight or flight' response. On the other hand, slow, deep breathing activates the parasympathetic nervous system, inducing a state of relaxation and calm. This is where the Vagus Nerve comes into play. It's a key component of the parasympathetic system and can be stimulated through specific breathing techniques, thereby impacting our overall state of well-being.

Deep breathing exercises stimulate the Vagus Nerve, which sends signals to the brain to slow down the heart rate and reduce blood pressure, fostering a state of calm. This activation of the Vagus Nerve is crucial for mental health, as it can reduce stress, anxiety, and depression symptoms. Moreover, controlled breathing can improve attention and increase emotional stability, making it an essential practice for a demographic deeply involved in high-stress professional environments and seeking balance in their hectic lives.

From a physiological standpoint, controlled breathing enhances respiratory efficiency. It increases oxygen exchange and can improve the capacity of the lungs. This increased efficiency not only boosts physical performance but also ensures better oxygen supply to the brain and other vital organs, enhancing overall health.

Furthermore, the science of breathing extends to its impact on the immune system. Regular practice of deep breathing exercises has been shown to strengthen the immune response, making the body more resilient to infections and diseases. This is particularly beneficial for individuals who are proactive about their health and well-being.

In the context of yoga and meditation, practices that are integral to the lifestyle of the target demographic, breathing plays a central role. These practices often incorporate specific breathing techniques (like pranayama in yoga) that are designed to stimulate the Vagus Nerve and promote mental clarity and physical well-being.

In summary, the science of breathing is a multifaceted field with far-reaching implications for health and wellness.

Understanding and harnessing the power of breathing can significantly impact one's quality of life, particularly in reducing stress, enhancing cognitive function, and improving physical health. For those immersed in a lifestyle that values wellness and self-improvement, incorporating controlled breathing techniques into daily routines can be a game-changer, offering a natural and effective way to stimulate the Vagus Nerve and achieve a state of balanced well-being.

# Step-by-step guided breathing exercises

Embarking on a journey to stimulate the Vagus Nerve through breathing requires understanding and practice. Here, we delve into step-by-step guided breathing exercises designed to activate this crucial nerve, fostering a sense of calm and improving overall mental and physical health. These exercises are particularly beneficial for individuals immersed in a demanding urban lifestyle, seeking to balance their hectic schedules with moments of tranquility and wellness.

## 1. Diaphragmatic Breathing

Begin by finding a comfortable, quiet space. Sit or lie down, placing one hand on your abdomen and the other on your chest.

This exercise involves deep breathing through the diaphragm, not shallow breathing from the chest.

Inhale slowly through your nose, counting to four. Feel your abdomen expand under your hand, while the hand on your chest remains relatively still.

Hold your breath for a count of two.

Exhale slowly through your mouth, counting to six. Focus on the hand on your abdomen, feeling it fall as you release the air.

Repeat this cycle for 5-10 minutes, focusing on the rhythm of your breathing.

## 2. 4-7-8 Breathing Technique

This technique, known for its simplicity and effectiveness, helps reduce anxiety and induce sleep.

Sit with your back straight. Place the tip of your tongue against the ridge of tissue behind your upper front teeth, keeping it there throughout the exercise.

Exhale completely through your mouth, making a whoosh sound.

Close your mouth and inhale quietly through your nose to a mental count of four.

Hold your breath for a count of seven.

Exhale completely through your mouth, making a whoosh sound to a count of eight.

This is one breath cycle. Repeat the cycle three more times for a total of four breaths.

## 3. Alternate Nostril Breathing

This exercise is commonly used in yoga and is known to calm the mind and balance the two hemispheres of the brain.

Sit comfortably with a straight spine. Rest your left hand on your lap.

With your right hand, use your thumb to close your right nostril.

Inhale slowly through your left nostril.

Close your left nostril with your fingers, then exhale through the right nostril.

Keep the left nostril closed, inhale through the right nostril.

Close the right nostril and exhale through the left. This completes one cycle.

Continue this pattern for 5 minutes, finishing with an exhale on the left side.

## 4. Progressive Relaxation Breath

This technique not only focuses on breathing but also on progressively relaxing each part of the body.

Lie down in a comfortable position. Close your eyes and take a few deep, slow breaths.

Beginning at your feet, tense them as you inhale deeply.

As you exhale, release all tension in your feet. Notice the sensation of relaxation.

Move progressively up the body – from your feet to your calves, thighs, abdomen, hands, arms, shoulders, neck, and face – repeating the process of tensing with inhalation and relaxing with exhalation.

Continue for 5-10 minutes, focusing on the rhythm of your breath and the sensation of relaxation.

These breathing exercises, when practiced regularly, can significantly impact your well-being. They are particularly effective for individuals in their 40s, living busy lives, yet seeking ways to maintain mental clarity and physical health. Integrating these practices into your daily routine, even for a few minutes, can provide a much-needed respite from the stresses of daily life, while also enhancing your body's natural relaxation response through Vagus Nerve stimulation.

# Customizing your breathing practice

Customizing your breathing practice to fit your unique lifestyle and needs is a crucial step towards enhancing the benefits of Vagus Nerve stimulation, especially for those living in a fast-paced urban environment with demanding careers. Tailoring these practices can significantly improve your mental clarity and physical well-being. To start, assess your daily schedule and identify the times when you feel most stressed. Are mornings hectic or do evenings bring a sense of anxiety? Recognizing these patterns helps you pinpoint the ideal moments for your breathing exercises, ensuring they seamlessly integrate into your day.

For instance, if mornings are typically rushed, a short, five-minute breathing exercise can set a calm tone for the day without adding to the chaos. Alternatively, if evenings are your time of stress, incorporating a relaxation technique before bed can aid in unwinding and promoting better sleep. It's essential to understand the different purposes of various breathing techniques. While diaphragmatic breathing is excellent for relaxation, alternate nostril breathing might be better suited for invigorating your mind and enhancing focus. Experiment with different methods to find what works best for you in various situations, and don't hesitate to adjust the exercises to accommodate any physical limitations, such as respiratory issues or back pain.

Incorporating mindfulness into your breathing exercises can further enhance their effectiveness. Being fully present, focusing on the sensation of each breath, strengthens the mind-body connection, leading to greater stress relief. Lastly, setting realistic goals for your practice and tracking your progress can be incredibly motivating. Whether it's dedicating five minutes each day to breathing exercises or incorporating them into your existing wellness routines, these small steps can lead to significant improvements in your overall well-being. Remember, the key to a successful breathing practice is consistency and personalization, ensuring that the exercises not only fit into your busy schedule but also cater to your individual needs and preferences.

# Chapter 4: The Power of Sound and Voice

## How sound impacts the vagus nerve

The intricate connection between sound and the Vagus Nerve is a subject of growing interest and importance, particularly for individuals immersed in the dynamic and often stressful environment of urban living. Sound, in its various forms, holds a profound influence on the Vagus Nerve, thereby impacting overall mental and physical well-being.

The Vagus Nerve, often described as the body's superhighway of communication, plays a pivotal role in the parasympathetic nervous system, which governs our body's 'rest and digest' responses. This nerve responds to a myriad of stimuli, including sound, which can either soothe or stimulate the nervous system. Understanding how sound impacts the Vagus Nerve is key to harnessing its potential for improving mental health and reducing stress.

When exposed to calming sounds, such as soft music, nature sounds, or the rhythmic hum of a chant, the Vagus Nerve is activated in a way that induces relaxation. This activation triggers a decrease in heart rate and blood pressure, fostering a state of calm and reducing stress levels. The mechanism behind this response involves the transmission of signals from the ear to the brain, which then communicates with the Vagus Nerve to initiate the relaxation response. This process exemplifies the body's remarkable ability to convert auditory signals into physiological changes.

Moreover, the type of sound and its characteristics play a crucial role in how the Vagus Nerve responds. Slow, melodious, and harmonious sounds tend to have a calming effect, while dissonant, loud, or abrupt sounds can trigger a stress response. For individuals in a fast-paced, urban setting, where noise pollution is common, finding respite in soothing sounds can be particularly beneficial.

The act of producing sound, such as humming, singing, or chanting, also has a direct impact on the Vagus Nerve. These activities involve the vibration of the vocal cords, which in turn stimulates the nerve. This kind of self-generated sound therapy can be an effective way to activate the Vagus Nerve. Humming, for instance, not only creates a soothing sound but also causes a physical vibration in the body, which enhances the nerve's stimulation. Similarly, singing, especially in a group setting, can increase vagal tone – the activity level of the Vagus Nerve – thereby improving emotional well-being and social connectivity.

Chanting, often used in meditation and yoga practices, combines the power of sound with rhythmic breathing, further enhancing the activation of the Vagus Nerve. The repetitive nature of chanting can lead to a meditative state, reducing stress and improving mental clarity. This practice is especially beneficial for individuals seeking holistic approaches to manage stress and improve mental health.

In conclusion, the impact of sound on the Vagus Nerve is a powerful tool in the quest for mental and physical well-being. Whether it's through listening to calming sounds or engaging in activities like humming, singing, or chanting, the ability to influence the Vagus Nerve through sound offers a natural and accessible means to reduce stress, improve emotional balance, and enhance overall health. For those living in an urban environment, integrating sound therapy into their wellness routine can be a simple yet effective way to combat the stresses of modern life, fostering a sense of peace and well-being amidst the chaos.

# Practical exercises involving humming, singing, and chanting

In the quest for holistic health, particularly for those navigating the complexities of urban life, practical exercises involving humming, singing, and chanting hold significant promise. These sound-based practices engage the Vagus Nerve, a key player in the body's relaxation response, offering a natural and accessible pathway to reduce stress, improve mental clarity, and enhance overall well-being.

**Humming: The Simplest Melody for Calm**

Humming is perhaps the most accessible form of sound therapy. It's a gentle, soothing practice that can be done anywhere, at any time, requiring no musical skill or training. The act of humming creates a physical vibration that resonates through the body, directly stimulating the Vagus Nerve.

*Basic Humming Exercise:*

Find a comfortable, quiet place.

Take a few deep breaths to relax.

Close your lips and begin to hum on an exhale, choosing a pitch that feels natural and soothing.

As you hum, focus on the vibrations in your chest and face.

Continue for 5-10 minutes, allowing the resonating sound to release tension and calm your mind.

**Singing: Elevating Wellness Through Song**

Singing, whether in a choir, in the shower, or along with your favorite songs, isn't just an enjoyable activity; it's a potent tool for stimulating the Vagus Nerve. Singing requires controlled breathing and engages the vocal cords, both of which activate the parasympathetic nervous system.

*Singing Exercise for Relaxation:*

Choose a song that you find uplifting and calming.

Focus on breathing deeply from your diaphragm as you sing.

Pay attention to the rhythm and flow of the melody, letting it guide your breath.

If comfortable, sing with others, as group singing can enhance the sense of connectedness and well-being.

**Chanting: A Rhythmic Path to Inner Peace**

Chanting, a staple in many spiritual and meditative practices, combines the power of rhythm and sound. It often incorporates meaningful phrases or mantras, enhancing its impact on mental clarity and focus.

*Chanting Exercise for Vagus Nerve Stimulation:*

Choose a mantra or phrase that resonates with you. It could be a single word like "peace" or a more extended chant.

Sit in a comfortable position, with your back straight.

Inhale deeply, and on the exhale, begin chanting your chosen mantra.

Feel the vibration of the sound in your throat and chest.

Continue for several minutes, allowing the rhythmic sound to bring a sense of calm and focus.

Each of these practices—humming, singing, and chanting—offers a unique pathway to engage the Vagus Nerve and tap into its power to relax the body and mind. For individuals in high-pressure environments, incorporating these exercises into daily routines can be transformative. They provide a moment of respite, a tool for managing stress, and a way to improve overall well-being without requiring significant time investment or resources. Furthermore, they align with interests in yoga, meditation, and holistic health, making them a perfect fit for individuals seeking natural, integrative approaches to wellness.

# Case studies: Transformation stories through sound therapy

The transformative power of sound therapy, particularly through practices like humming, singing, and chanting, is vividly illustrated in several case studies. These stories showcase the profound impact sound therapy can have on individuals from various walks of life, particularly those who are part of a demographic characterized by high-stress urban living.

### Case Study 1: The Stressed Executive

Mark, a 42-year-old executive in a high-pressure finance job, struggled with chronic stress and insomnia. His busy lifestyle in the bustling city left him little time for relaxation. After attending a workshop on sound therapy, Mark began incorporating daily humming exercises into his routine. He would hum for ten minutes during his morning commute, using the vibrations to calm his mind. Over several weeks, Mark noticed a significant decrease in his stress levels. His sleep improved, and he reported feeling more centered and focused at work. The simple act of humming had activated his Vagus Nerve, promoting a state of calm and reducing his anxiety.

## Case Study 2: The Yoga Enthusiast

Sarah, a 38-year-old yoga instructor, experienced bouts of anxiety and mood swings. Despite her active lifestyle, she found herself overwhelmed by the pressures of running her own studio. Sarah started integrating chanting into her daily meditation practice, focusing on mantras that promoted peace and stability. The chanting not only deepened her meditation experience but also had a profound calming effect on her nervous system. Over time, Sarah's anxiety levels decreased, and she reported a more consistent mood pattern. The rhythmic chanting had effectively stimulated her Vagus Nerve, enhancing her emotional well-being.

## Case Study 3: The Retired Veteran

John, a 60-year-old retired military veteran, suffered from PTSD and related sleep disturbances. Traditional therapies had offered limited relief. He was introduced to sound therapy as part of a holistic wellness program. John began participating in group singing sessions, which were therapeutic and community-building. Singing in a group helped John feel more connected and less isolated. The act of singing regulated his breathing and activated his Vagus Nerve, which significantly reduced his symptoms of PTSD and improved his sleep quality.

## Case Study 4: The Busy Mother

Emily, a 35-year-old mother of two, juggled her career and family responsibilities, leading to high levels of stress and occasional anxiety attacks. She started practicing guided sound meditation, focusing on deep breathing combined with soft humming. This practice became her nightly routine, helping her unwind and relax after a long day. The humming exercises helped in regulating her heart rate and calming her mind, providing her with a tool to manage her stress and anxiety effectively.

These case studies demonstrate the diverse applications and benefits of sound therapy through humming, singing, and chanting. Each story highlights how individuals, despite their different backgrounds and challenges, found relief and transformation through the simple yet powerful practice of sound therapy. This approach, especially pertinent to those living in high-stress environments, offers an accessible, natural method to stimulate the Vagus Nerve, promoting mental clarity, emotional stability, and overall well-being.

# Chapter 5: Physical Exercises for Mind and Body Harmony

## Tailored exercises for vagus nerve stimulation

Tailoring exercises for the stimulation of the Vagus Nerve is a vital strategy for enhancing mental and physical well-being, particularly for individuals immersed in the demanding rhythms of urban life. These exercises, by activating the Vagus Nerve, play a crucial role in regulating the body's relaxation response, thereby promoting a state of calm and balance which is essential for health and wellness.

The Vagus Nerve, a key element of the parasympathetic nervous system, orchestrates the body's relaxation response. It works to lower the heart rate, reduce blood pressure, and decrease stress hormones. Exercises that effectively stimulate this nerve can have a significant impact on stress and anxiety reduction, heart health improvement, and overall well-being enhancement. The beauty of these exercises lies in their adaptability and accessibility, allowing individuals from all walks of life to incorporate them into their daily routines.

For individuals leading a fast-paced urban lifestyle, often characterized by high stress and limited time, integrating Vagus Nerve stimulating exercises can be both a necessity and a challenge. These exercises range from simple breathing techniques to more physical activities like yoga or light aerobic exercises. The key is to engage in movements that encourage deep and rhythmic breathing, which in turn activates the Vagus Nerve. Activities such as slow-paced yoga, tai chi, or even leisurely walks in nature can be incredibly effective. They not only stimulate the nerve but also provide an opportunity for mindfulness and mental clarity.

The practice of deep, diaphragmatic breathing during these activities is particularly effective. This type of breathing encourages a full oxygen exchange – beneficial for the heart and blood pressure, and by extension, it stimulates the Vagus Nerve. Yoga, with its emphasis on breath control and gentle movements, stands out as a particularly effective practice for Vagus Nerve stimulation. The combination of breathing, stretching, and mindful presence that yoga entails can significantly reduce stress levels and promote a sense of inner peace.

Moreover, incorporating these exercises into a daily routine doesn't require drastic changes. It can be as simple as dedicating a few minutes each morning to deep breathing exercises, taking a short walk during lunch breaks, or practicing a series of yoga poses before bed. The goal is to create a routine that feels less like a task and more like a rejuvenating break, a moment in the day dedicated entirely to personal well-being.

In conclusion, exercises that stimulate the Vagus Nerve are a powerful tool in the quest for improved mental and physical health. They offer a natural and effective way to combat the stresses of modern life, especially for those in high-pressure urban environments. By engaging in these exercises regularly, individuals can experience significant improvements in their stress levels, mental clarity, and overall health, leading to a more balanced and fulfilling lifestyle.

# Incorporating movement into your daily routine

Incorporating movement into your daily routine is an essential strategy for enhancing overall mental and physical harmony, particularly for individuals leading busy, high-stress urban lives. Movement, in various forms, not only improves physical health but also significantly impacts mental well-being, acting as a natural stimulant for the Vagus Nerve and thus promoting relaxation and stress reduction.

In the fast-paced rhythm of modern urban life, finding time for structured exercise can be challenging. However, integrating movement into your daily routine doesn't necessarily require large blocks of time or significant lifestyle changes. It's about finding small, manageable ways to incorporate more physical activity into your everyday life.

Start with identifying opportunities within your current daily schedule where movement can be seamlessly included. This could be as simple as opting to take the stairs instead of the elevator, parking a little further from your office to allow for a short walk, or even standing and stretching during breaks at work. These small increments of activity can accumulate to a significant amount of physical exercise over time, contributing to your overall health and stimulating the Vagus Nerve.

For those who spend a lot of time sitting, particularly in office environments, setting reminders to stand and stretch every hour can be beneficial. Incorporating stretching exercises, especially those that open up the chest and involve deep breathing, can activate the Vagus Nerve, promoting relaxation and reducing stress. Simple stretches, like reaching the arms overhead or gentle neck rolls, can be done almost anywhere and require only a minute or two.

Lunch breaks offer another opportunity for movement. A brisk walk outside not only provides physical exercise but also offers a mental break, allowing you to return to your afternoon tasks with renewed energy and focus. If possible, walking meetings can be a novel way to combine work and movement, particularly in a collaborative, dynamic work environment.

For individuals who enjoy hobbies like yoga and meditation, integrating these practices into your routine can be particularly effective. Yoga, with its combination of physical poses, controlled breathing, and meditation, is an excellent way to stimulate the Vagus Nerve. Even a short, 10-minute yoga session in the morning or evening can have significant benefits for both mind and body.

Weekends and leisure time provide additional opportunities for incorporating more intensive physical activities, such as hiking, cycling, or participating in group sports. These activities not only improve physical fitness but also provide social interaction and mental relaxation, further enhancing the stimulation of the Vagus Nerve and promoting overall well-being.

In conclusion, integrating movement into your daily routine is a practical and effective way to enhance your physical and mental health. By finding ways to include more activity in your day-to-day life, you can improve your Vagus Nerve function, reduce stress, and achieve a greater sense of balance and harmony. This approach is particularly beneficial for busy individuals seeking holistic methods to improve their health and well-being amidst the demands of urban living.

# Part III: Overcoming Challenges

# Chapter 6: Addressing and Alleviating Anxiety

## Understanding the anxiety-vagus nerve connection

Understanding the complex relationship between anxiety and the Vagus Nerve is vital for individuals, especially those immersed in the demanding urban lifestyle, seeking effective ways to manage anxiety. The Vagus Nerve, a key component of the body's autonomic nervous system, plays a significant role in regulating our stress responses. It acts as the body's natural calming agent, counteracting the sympathetic nervous system's "fight or flight" response and helping to maintain a balance in the nervous system. This balance is crucial for reducing anxiety levels and promoting relaxation.

Anxiety often presents as a heightened state of arousal, a byproduct of an overactive sympathetic nervous system. This heightened state can lead to various physical symptoms like an increased heart rate, rapid breathing, and heightened alertness. While these are natural responses to perceived threats, persistent symptoms can lead to chronic anxiety, significantly impacting one's daily life and overall well-being. The Vagus Nerve, through its influence on the parasympathetic nervous system, works to mitigate these responses. Stimulating this nerve can induce a relaxation response, reducing the physical symptoms associated with anxiety.

The concept of 'vagal tone,' which refers to the activity level of the Vagus Nerve, is crucial in this context. High vagal tone is associated with a better ability to regulate stress responses and is linked to improved mood and reduced anxiety. Conversely, low vagal tone often correlates with increased stress and anxiety levels. Therefore, enhancing one's vagal tone is a key strategy in managing anxiety effectively.

There are various methods to stimulate the Vagus Nerve, thereby improving vagal tone and reducing anxiety. Deep, diaphragmatic breathing is one of the simplest and most effective methods. This type of breathing encourages a full oxygen exchange and triggers the Vagus Nerve, promoting a state of calmness. Additionally, practices such as yoga and meditation, which combine physical postures with deep breathing, are excellent for stimulating the Vagus Nerve. They not only help in reducing the immediate symptoms of anxiety but also contribute to long-term emotional regulation and stress management.

Moreover, integrating mindfulness practices into daily life can enhance the effectiveness of these techniques. Being present and aware during yoga or breathing exercises can deepen the relaxation response and further reduce anxiety levels. For individuals leading busy urban lives, finding time for such practices can be challenging. However, incorporating short, manageable sessions of deep breathing or yoga into the daily routine can be highly beneficial. Even a few minutes of focused breathing or mindful movement each day can contribute significantly to reducing anxiety and improving overall well-being.

In summary, understanding the anxiety-Vagus Nerve connection is integral to developing effective strategies for anxiety management. By recognizing the importance of the Vagus Nerve in regulating stress responses and implementing practices to stimulate this nerve, individuals can significantly improve their ability to manage anxiety. This approach, focusing on enhancing vagal tone through practices like deep breathing, yoga, and mindfulness, offers a holistic and effective way to combat anxiety, especially for those in high-stress urban environments.

# Practical strategies and exercises for anxiety relief

In addressing anxiety, practical strategies and exercises play a pivotal role, offering those affected a pathway to relief and improved well-being. For individuals living in a high-paced urban environment, dealing with the pressures of a demanding career and personal life, anxiety can be a significant challenge. Implementing effective strategies for anxiety relief is not just beneficial but essential for maintaining a balanced life.

## Breathing Techniques for Anxiety Relief

Breathing exercises are among the most effective methods for managing anxiety. They can be performed anywhere and require no special equipment, making them highly accessible for anyone, regardless of their lifestyle or schedule.

**Diaphragmatic Breathing:** This involves deep breathing from the belly rather than shallow breathing from the chest. Practicing diaphragmatic breathing for just a few minutes daily can trigger the relaxation response, reducing anxiety levels.

**4-7-8 Breathing Technique:** This technique, developed by Dr. Andrew Weil, is simple yet powerful. It involves inhaling for

4 seconds, holding the breath for 7 seconds, and exhaling for 8 seconds. This pattern helps slow down the heart rate and induces a state of calm.

## Mindfulness and Meditation for Anxiety

Mindfulness and meditation are proven methods for reducing anxiety. They involve focusing the mind on the present moment, which helps break the cycle of worry and stress.

**Mindful Breathing:** Focusing on the breath helps anchor the mind in the present moment, providing a break from anxious thoughts.

**Guided Meditation:** Using guided meditation apps or online resources can be a helpful way to start a meditation practice. These guides often include instructions for relaxation and visualization techniques tailored to relieve anxiety.

## Physical Exercise for Stress Relief

Physical activity is a potent antidote to anxiety. It not only improves physical health but also releases endorphins, natural mood lifters that can reduce stress and anxiety.

**Yoga**: Incorporating yoga into your routine can be particularly beneficial. The combination of physical postures, controlled breathing, and meditation in yoga provides a holistic approach to managing anxiety.

**Aerobic Exercise:** Activities like walking, running, cycling, or swimming, especially performed outdoors, can significantly reduce anxiety levels.

## Cognitive Behavioral Techniques

Cognitive Behavioral Therapy (CBT) techniques can also be effective in managing anxiety. These involve identifying and challenging negative thought patterns and replacing them with more positive, realistic ones.

**Journaling:** Writing down your thoughts and feelings can provide an outlet for expressing anxiety and identifying triggers.

**Cognitive Reframing:** This involves identifying negative thoughts and consciously replacing them with positive or realistic ones.

## Lifestyle Changes

Making specific lifestyle changes can also help manage anxiety levels.

**Regular Sleep Patterns:** Establishing a regular sleep pattern can significantly affect anxiety levels. Lack of sleep can exacerbate anxiety, so aiming for 7-9 hours of quality sleep is crucial.

**Balanced Diet:** A diet rich in fruits, vegetables, whole grains, and lean proteins can support overall health and reduce symptoms of anxiety.

## Relaxation Techniques

Relaxation techniques such as progressive muscle relaxation or biofeedback can help in reducing anxiety. These methods involve learning to relax muscles in the body, which can help ease anxiety symptoms.

**Progressive Muscle Relaxation:** This technique involves tensing and relaxing different muscle groups in the body, which can help reduce the physical symptoms of anxiety.

**Biofeedback**: Using sensors that measure bodily functions like heart rate and muscle tension, biofeedback teaches how to control these responses, helping to reduce anxiety.

In conclusion, various practical strategies and exercises can effectively relieve anxiety. From breathing techniques and meditation to physical exercise and cognitive behavioral methods, these approaches offer a comprehensive toolkit for managing anxiety. For individuals in high-stress environments, incorporating these practices into their daily routine can make a significant difference in their overall quality of life, leading to reduced anxiety and improved mental and physical well-being.

# Success stories of overcoming anxiety

Success stories of overcoming anxiety are both inspiring and illuminating, particularly for those who grapple with the fast-paced, high-pressure demands of urban living. These narratives not only showcase the resilience of individuals but also highlight the effectiveness of various strategies in managing and alleviating anxiety. Here, we delve into a series of transformative journeys that underscore the triumph of the human spirit over anxiety.

**The Corporate Executive's Journey to Calm**

Michael, a 45-year-old corporate executive, faced intense pressure in his high-stakes job. Long hours and constant deadlines led to chronic anxiety, affecting his performance and personal life. Michael's journey began with acknowledging his anxiety and seeking help. He started practicing mindfulness meditation every morning, focusing on deep breathing and present moment awareness. Over time, this practice helped him gain perspective on his stressors and respond to them more calmly. Michael also incorporated regular aerobic exercise into his routine, which not only improved his physical health but also provided a mental break from work-related stress. Through these combined efforts, Michael experienced a significant reduction in his anxiety levels, regained his focus at work, and found more joy in his personal life.

## The Young Mother's Path to Peace

Emma, a 38-year-old mother of two, struggled with postpartum anxiety. The demands of motherhood, coupled with sleep deprivation, left her feeling constantly on edge. Emma's turning point came when she joined a yoga class designed for new mothers. The physical postures, combined with controlled breathing, helped in easing her tense muscles and calming her mind. She also found solace in the supportive community of other mothers. Additionally, Emma began writing in a journal, a practice that allowed her to express her feelings and fears in a safe, private space. Gradually, Emma's anxiety became more manageable, allowing her to enjoy motherhood more fully.

**The Artist's Creative Escape**

Alex, a 30-year-old graphic designer and artist, battled anxiety that stifled his creativity. Overwhelmed by client demands and creative blocks, Alex felt his anxiety spiraling. He decided to tackle it by changing his environment and routine. Alex started taking long walks in nature, using this time to disconnect from digital devices and reconnect with his surroundings. He also experimented with sound therapy, particularly with calming nature sounds and music during his work. These changes not only provided Alex with much-needed mental clarity but also reignited his creative spark, leading to a newfound enthusiasm for his work and artistic projects.

**The Retiree's Newfound Freedom**

Susan, a 65-year-old retiree, experienced heightened anxiety during the transition out of her long-standing career. The sudden change in routine and loss of a familiar structure led to feelings of unease and worry. Susan found relief through volunteering, which gave her a sense of purpose and community connection. She also enrolled in a Tai Chi class, a gentle form of exercise that emphasized slow movements and deep breathing, ideal for her age and fitness level. These activities not only helped Susan in managing her anxiety but also brought new friendships and experiences into her life, enriching her retirement years.

Each of these stories is a testament to the power of taking proactive steps to manage anxiety. Whether it's through mindfulness, physical exercise, journaling, or changing one's routine, these individuals demonstrate that anxiety can be alleviated and that a more balanced, fulfilling life is achievable. Their journeys offer hope and practical insights for anyone facing anxiety, especially those in similar urban, high-pressure environments, showing that with the right strategies and support, overcoming anxiety is not just a possibility but a reality.

# Chapter 7: Conquering Chronic Stress

## The impact of chronic stress on the vagus nerve

The impact of chronic stress on the Vagus Nerve is a critical aspect of understanding how stress affects our overall health and well-being, particularly for individuals in a fast-paced, high-stress urban environment. Chronic stress, a common feature of modern life, especially in high-demand settings, can have profound and lasting effects on the Vagus Nerve, thereby impacting the body's ability to maintain balance and resilience.

### Understanding the Vagus Nerve

The Vagus Nerve, one of the longest nerves in the body, is a fundamental part of the parasympathetic nervous system, often referred to as the "rest and digest" system. It plays a vital role in regulating many of the body's key functions, including heart rate, digestion, and immune response. The health and functionality of the Vagus Nerve are paramount in managing stress effectively.

## Chronic Stress and the Vagus Nerve

When the body is exposed to acute stress, it triggers the "fight or flight" response, a survival mechanism that prepares the body to respond to immediate threats. However, in the case of chronic stress, this response is continuously activated, putting excessive strain on the body, including the Vagus Nerve. Over time, this can lead to a decrease in vagal tone, the activity level of the Vagus Nerve, which is essential for calming the body after stress.

Low vagal tone is associated with various health issues, including heart problems, gastrointestinal issues, and mental health disorders like depression and anxiety. Chronic stress can lead to a persistent state of heightened nervous system arousal, making it harder for the Vagus Nerve to effectively perform its role in calming the body, thereby exacerbating these health issues.

## Physical Implications of Chronic Stress on the Vagus Nerve

The physical implications of chronic stress on the Vagus Nerve are manifold. High-stress levels can lead to an increased heart rate and elevated blood pressure, straining the cardiovascular system. The digestive system, too, is significantly affected, as the Vagus Nerve plays a key role in regulating digestive processes. Chronic stress can disrupt digestion, leading to issues like irritable bowel syndrome (IBS), indigestion, and acid reflux.

Moreover, the Vagus Nerve influences the immune system. Prolonged stress can weaken the nerve's ability to regulate immune responses, making the body more susceptible to infections and illnesses. It also affects respiratory functions, which can exacerbate conditions like asthma and chronic obstructive pulmonary disease (COPD).

## Mental and Emotional Impact

On a mental and emotional level, the impaired function of the Vagus Nerve due to chronic stress can have significant repercussions. It can lead to heightened anxiety, depression, and mood swings. The inability to relax due to low vagal tone can create a cycle of continuous stress, affecting sleep patterns, concentration, and overall mental clarity.

**Coping with Chronic Stress**

To counter the effects of chronic stress on the Vagus Nerve, it's crucial to adopt strategies that enhance vagal tone and promote relaxation. Practices like deep breathing exercises, meditation, and yoga are highly effective in stimulating the Vagus Nerve. Engaging in regular physical exercise, maintaining a healthy diet, and ensuring adequate sleep are also key in supporting the nerve's health.

Moreover, activities that promote positive social interactions and emotional connections, such as spending time with loved ones or engaging in community activities, can boost vagal tone. These activities stimulate the release of oxytocin, often referred to as the "love hormone," which has a calming effect on the Vagus Nerve.

In conclusion, understanding the impact of chronic stress on the Vagus Nerve is essential for individuals seeking to maintain a balanced and healthy lifestyle amidst the pressures of modern living. By adopting holistic approaches that focus on enhancing vagal tone and reducing stress, it's possible to mitigate the adverse effects of chronic stress and improve overall health and well-being. This approach is not only beneficial for immediate stress relief but also for building long-term resilience against future stressors.

# Holistic approaches to stress management

Holistic approaches to stress management encompass a comprehensive view of dealing with chronic stress, particularly significant for individuals leading complex, high-demand urban lives. These approaches do not merely focus on alleviating the symptoms of stress but aim to address its root causes, integrating physical, mental, emotional, and environmental aspects to promote overall well-being.

## Understanding Holistic Stress Management

Holistic stress management is grounded in the understanding that stress is not just a mental or physical state but a condition influenced by a variety of factors including lifestyle, environment, emotional well-being, and social interactions. This approach seeks to create a balanced life where stressors are not just managed but are also significantly reduced through various techniques and lifestyle changes.

## Physical Dimension: Diet, Exercise, and Sleep

The physical dimension of stress management involves taking care of the body through diet, exercise, and sleep - fundamental aspects that directly impact stress levels.

Diet: Consuming a balanced diet rich in fruits, vegetables, whole grains, lean protein, and healthy fats can provide the necessary nutrients to combat the effects of stress. Limiting caffeine and sugar intake is also crucial as they can exacerbate anxiety and stress.

Exercise: Regular physical activity is a powerful stress reliever. Activities like brisk walking, running, yoga, or swimming not only improve physical health but also release endorphins, natural mood lifters. Exercise also helps in improving sleep quality, another critical factor in managing stress.

Sleep: Adequate sleep is essential for overall health and stress management. Establishing a regular sleep routine, creating a comfortable sleep environment, and avoiding screen time before bed can enhance sleep quality.

## Mental and Emotional Dimension: Mindfulness and Cognitive Techniques

Mental and emotional well-being is central to handling stress. Mindfulness practices and cognitive techniques can significantly reduce stress levels by altering thought patterns and enhancing emotional resilience.

Mindfulness and Meditation: Practices like mindfulness meditation, deep breathing exercises, and progressive muscle relaxation can help in calming the mind and reducing the physiological effects of stress. They encourage a state of present moment awareness and relaxation.

Cognitive Behavioral Therapy (CBT): CBT is an effective method for managing stress by changing negative thought patterns and developing more positive coping mechanisms.

## Social and Environmental Dimension: Building Support Networks

Social interactions and environmental factors play a significant role in stress management. Building a supportive social network and creating a stress-free environment are key components of a holistic approach.

Social Support: Strong relationships with family, friends, and community can provide emotional support and a sense of belonging, crucial in times of stress.

Environmental Changes: Creating a peaceful and organized living and working environment can reduce stress triggers. This includes managing noise levels, ensuring adequate lighting, and maintaining a clutter-free space.

## Personal Development and Hobbies: Engaging in Fulfilling Activities

Engaging in activities that bring joy and fulfillment is an essential aspect of holistic stress management. Hobbies, personal development, and leisure activities provide an outlet for creativity and relaxation.

Hobbies: Pursuing hobbies like gardening, painting, cooking, or playing a musical instrument can be therapeutic and provide a break from routine stressors.

Personal Development: Attending workshops, seminars, or engaging in activities that promote personal growth can enhance self-esteem and provide tools for managing stress.

## Integrating Holistic Practices into Daily Life

Successfully integrating these holistic practices into daily life involves creating a balanced routine that accommodates physical, mental, and emotional well-being. This might include setting aside time for exercise, practicing meditation daily, engaging in social activities, and ensuring a balanced diet and adequate sleep. It also involves being mindful of one's environment and making necessary changes to promote a stress-free atmosphere.

In conclusion, holistic approaches to stress management offer a comprehensive way to not only manage stress but to enhance overall quality of life. By addressing the physical, mental, emotional, social, and environmental factors that contribute to stress, individuals can develop a more balanced, healthier approach to life, particularly crucial for those in high-stress urban settings. This multifaceted approach not only helps in alleviating current stress but also builds resilience against future stressors.

# Building resilience against future stress

Building resilience against future stress is a fundamental aspect of maintaining long-term health and well-being, particularly for individuals navigating the complexities of urban, high-stress environments. Resilience, the ability to bounce back from stressful situations, is not an innate trait but a skill that can be developed and strengthened over time. This chapter delves into various strategies and practices that help build resilience, enabling individuals to better handle future stressors and maintain a balanced life.

## Understanding Resilience

Resilience is often misunderstood as the ability to endure stress without any impact. In reality, resilience is about adaptive coping, learning from stressors, and emerging stronger and more capable. It involves recognizing the effects of stress on one's life and taking proactive steps to manage it effectively. Building resilience is a continuous process that requires dedication and practice.

A resilient mindset begins with a positive but realistic outlook on life. It involves recognizing that while stress is a part of life, it does not define one's entire existence. Cultivating a growth mindset, where challenges are seen as opportunities for growth rather than insurmountable obstacles, is crucial. This mindset can be fostered through practices like mindfulness, cognitive reframing, and maintaining a sense of purpose and meaning in life.

## Mindfulness and Emotional Regulation

Mindfulness, the practice of being present and fully engaged with the current moment, is a powerful tool for building resilience. It helps in recognizing and accepting one's emotional responses to stress without being overwhelmed by them. Techniques like mindful breathing, meditation, and yoga can enhance emotional regulation, providing a solid foundation for resilience.

## Physical Health as a Pillar of Resilience

Physical health plays a vital role in building resilience against stress. Regular physical activity, a nutritious diet, and adequate sleep are essential components. Exercise not only improves physical strength and endurance but also reduces the impact of stress on the body. A balanced diet provides the necessary nutrients to fuel the body and mind, while sufficient sleep is crucial for recovery and mental clarity.

Also, strong social connections are a key component of resilience. Building and maintaining supportive relationships provide emotional support and a sense of belonging. Engaging in community activities, nurturing friendships, and seeking support when needed can bolster one's ability to cope with stress.

## Stress Management Techniques

Learning and regularly practicing stress management techniques can prepare individuals to handle future stressors more effectively. Techniques such as deep breathing exercises, progressive muscle relaxation, and guided imagery can be incorporated into daily routines to help manage stress responses.

Resilience involves adapting to change and uncertainty, skills particularly relevant in the fast-paced modern world. Developing flexibility in thinking and behavior helps in navigating unforeseen challenges. Embracing change as a part of life and finding ways to adapt can significantly enhance resilience.

## Setting Boundaries and Self-Care

Setting healthy boundaries in personal and professional life is essential for maintaining resilience. Understanding and respecting one's limits helps prevent burnout and chronic stress. Additionally, prioritizing self-care and taking time for activities that bring joy and relaxation are important for replenishing one's mental and emotional energy.

Building resilience is an ongoing journey that involves reflective practices and continuous learning. Regularly reflecting on past experiences, identifying lessons learned, and applying them to future situations can enhance one's ability to cope with stress. This reflective process encourages continuous personal growth and development.

In conclusion, building resilience against future stress is a multifaceted approach that encompasses mental, emotional, physical, and social aspects. By developing a resilient mindset, prioritizing physical health, nurturing social connections, practicing effective stress management techniques, adapting to change, setting boundaries, and engaging in reflective practices, individuals can equip themselves with the tools necessary to handle future stressors more effectively. This approach not only helps in managing stress but also contributes to a more fulfilling and balanced life, especially for those in high-pressure urban settings.

# Part IV: Advanced Techniques

# Chapter 8: Dietary Impacts on the Vagus Nerve

## Foods that stimulate and inhibit the vagus nerve

The connection between diet and the Vagus Nerve is a vital component in the context of managing chronic stress and overall well-being. The Vagus Nerve, a central part of the body's relaxation response system, can be influenced significantly by what we eat. Certain foods can stimulate this nerve, enhancing its function and promoting a state of calm, while others can have an inhibitory effect, potentially contributing to stress and related health issues.

### Foods That Stimulate the Vagus Nerve

Certain foods and nutrients are known to positively influence the activity of the Vagus Nerve.

**Omega-3 Fatty Acids:** Found in fish like salmon, mackerel, and sardines, omega-3 fatty acids are essential for brain health and have been shown to increase vagal tone, thereby promoting relaxation and reducing stress levels.

**Probiotics**: These beneficial bacteria, found in fermented foods like yogurt, kefir, sauerkraut, and kombucha, can improve gut health. A healthy gut is linked to better Vagus Nerve function, as this nerve plays a key role in the gut-brain axis.

**Leafy Greens and Vegetables:** Rich in vitamins and minerals, leafy greens like spinach, kale, and swiss chard, and other vegetables support overall health and are beneficial for the Vagus Nerve. Magnesium, found in these foods, is particularly effective in supporting nerve function.

**Fruits**: Fruits like blueberries, strawberries, and oranges, rich in antioxidants and vitamins, can help reduce inflammation in the body, supporting vagal activity.

**Nuts and Seeds**: Almonds, walnuts, flaxseeds, and chia seeds are excellent sources of nutrients that support nerve health and reduce inflammation.

**Lean Proteins:** Sources of lean protein, such as chicken, turkey, and legumes, provide the amino acids necessary for neurotransmitter production, which is crucial for Vagus Nerve function.

**Foods That Inhibit the Vagus Nerve**

Just as some foods can stimulate the Vagus Nerve, others can have an inhibitory effect, potentially leading to decreased vagal tone and increased stress.

**Processed and Sugary Foods:** High intake of processed foods, sugars, and refined carbohydrates can lead to inflammation and oxidative stress, which may negatively impact the Vagus Nerve.

**Excessive Caffeine and Alcohol:** While moderate consumption might not have a significant impact, excessive intake of caffeine and alcohol can disrupt the balance of neurotransmitters and potentially inhibit the Vagus Nerve.

**Trans Fats and High-Fat Processed Foods:** These can contribute to poor cardiovascular health, which in turn, can impact vagal tone negatively.

**Implementing a Vagus Nerve-Friendly Diet**

Incorporating a Vagus Nerve-friendly diet involves focusing on whole, nutrient-rich foods while minimizing the intake of processed foods, excessive sugars, and unhealthy fats. A balanced diet that includes a variety of fruits, vegetables, lean proteins, healthy fats, and fermented foods can support the overall function of the Vagus Nerve.

For those living in urban environments and dealing with the stresses of modern life, paying attention to diet can be a powerful tool in managing stress and enhancing well-being. It's not about strict dietary restrictions but about making mindful choices that support overall health and the optimal functioning of the Vagus Nerve.

In conclusion, understanding the dietary impacts on the Vagus Nerve is essential for anyone looking to manage stress effectively and improve their overall health. By focusing on foods that stimulate the Vagus Nerve and avoiding those that inhibit it, individuals can take a significant step towards building resilience against stress and enhancing their quality of life. This approach to diet, combined with other stress management techniques, forms a comprehensive strategy for addressing chronic stress and promoting long-term well-being.

# A 30-day meal plan for optimal nerve function

Creating a 30-day meal plan aimed at enhancing the optimal function of the Vagus Nerve involves incorporating foods that stimulate this vital nerve while avoiding those that might inhibit its function. This meal plan is designed for individuals living in a high-stress urban environment, looking to balance their hectic lifestyle with a diet that supports their mental and physical well-being.

**Week 1: Establishing a Healthy Foundation**

*Day 1-7: Focus on introducing Omega-3 rich foods, probiotics, and plenty of fruits and vegetables.*

**Breakfast**: Start with a smoothie made from spinach, blueberries, flaxseed, and almond milk. This combination provides antioxidants, Omega-3s, and fiber.

**Lunch**: Opt for a salad with mixed greens, salmon (rich in Omega-3), avocados, nuts, and a light olive oil dressing.

**Dinner**: Prepare a stir-fry with lean chicken, a variety of vegetables like bell peppers and broccoli, and brown rice.

**Snacks**: Include Greek yogurt and a handful of almonds or walnuts.

**Week 2: Enhancing Gut Health**

*Day 8-14: Incorporate more probiotic and prebiotic foods to improve gut health, which is crucial for Vagus Nerve function.*

**Breakfast**: Yogurt with a sprinkle of chia seeds and fresh fruit.

**Lunch**: A quinoa bowl with fermented vegetables like kimchi or sauerkraut, leafy greens, and a source of lean protein like grilled tofu.

**Dinner**: Grilled fish with a side of asparagus and sweet potatoes.

**Snacks**: Carrot and celery sticks with hummus, and a piece of fruit.

**Week 3: Focus on Anti-Inflammatory Foods**

*Day 15-21: Emphasize foods that reduce inflammation, which can impact the Vagus Nerve.*

**Breakfast**: Oatmeal with turmeric, a dash of black pepper, and berries.

**Lunch**: Spinach salad with grilled chicken, avocado, tomatoes, and a dressing made from extra virgin olive oil and lemon.

**Dinner**: Baked salmon with a side of quinoa and steamed vegetables like broccoli or Brussels sprouts.

**Snacks**: A handful of berries or mixed nuts, and green tea.

**Week 4: Consolidating Healthy Eating Habits**

*Day 22-30: Continue with a balanced diet focusing on whole foods, lean proteins, and healthy fats.*

**Breakfast**: Scrambled eggs with spinach and whole-grain toast.

**Lunch**: Whole grain wrap with turkey, avocado, lettuce, and mustard. Serve with a side of mixed greens.

**Dinner**: Grilled shrimp with a medley of roasted vegetables like bell peppers, zucchini, and eggplant.

**Snacks**: Yogurt with a sprinkle of flaxseed, or apple slices with almond butter.

Throughout the 30 days, hydration should be a priority. Aim for at least 8 glasses of water per day. Herbal teas like chamomile or ginger can also be included. Practicing mindful eating – taking time to savor and enjoy each meal – is also crucial. This practice helps in reducing stress and improving digestion, further benefiting the Vagus Nerve.

The key to this meal plan is moderation and variety. It's important to include a wide range of foods to ensure all nutrients are covered. Occasional indulgences are fine, as long as the overall diet remains balanced and focused on whole, unprocessed foods.

In conclusion, this 30-day meal plan is designed not just to nourish the body but also to support the optimal function of the Vagus Nerve. By focusing on nutrient-rich foods that stimulate the nerve and reduce inflammation, and by adopting healthy eating habits, individuals can significantly enhance their body's ability to manage stress. This holistic approach to diet, combined with other lifestyle modifications, can lead to improved mental clarity, reduced anxiety, and a more balanced and fulfilling life.

# The role of hydration and nutrition

The integral roles of hydration and nutrition in the optimal functioning of the Vagus Nerve are essential considerations for maintaining balance and well-being, especially in the context of a fast-paced urban lifestyle. Adequate hydration and a balanced diet are crucial in ensuring the health and proper functioning of the Vagus Nerve, a key player in managing stress and emotional regulation.

Water, the most fundamental element for bodily functions, is vital for the health of the Vagus Nerve. Every cell in the body, including nerve cells, relies on proper hydration to function effectively. Staying adequately hydrated ensures that the electrolyte balance necessary for nerve signal transmission is maintained. Dehydration can lead to a decrease in vagal tone, potentially increasing stress and anxiety levels. The recommended daily water intake is around 8-10 glasses, equivalent to approximately 2 liters, though this can vary based on factors like climate and physical activity. Signs of dehydration, such as dry mouth, fatigue, headache, and dizziness, can have adverse effects on nerve function and overall health. Therefore, it's crucial, particularly for urban dwellers who might face a hectic lifestyle, to ensure they are consistently well-hydrated.

Beyond hydration, nutrition plays a pivotal role in the functioning of the Vagus Nerve. A balanced diet, rich in fruits, vegetables, whole grains, lean proteins, and healthy fats, provides the necessary nutrients that support nerve health. Foods rich in Omega-3 fatty acids, such as fish, nuts, and seeds, are particularly beneficial as they enhance the nerve's function and improve its tone. Antioxidant-rich foods like berries and leafy greens help combat inflammation in the body, which can positively impact the Vagus Nerve. Conversely, a diet high in processed foods, sugars, and unhealthy fats can have the opposite effect, leading to increased inflammation and reduced vagal tone.

Moreover, specific nutrients play direct roles in supporting the Vagus Nerve. Magnesium, found in foods like spinach, nuts, and whole grains, is crucial for nerve function. Probiotics, which improve gut health, also benefit the Vagus Nerve, as there is a significant connection between the gut and the brain via this nerve. Fermented foods like yogurt and sauerkraut are excellent sources of probiotics.

Incorporating a diet that supports the Vagus Nerve is not just about adding certain foods; it's also about adopting a holistic approach to eating. This includes mindful eating practices, where the focus is on savoring and enjoying meals without distractions, which can enhance digestion and reduce stress. Additionally, for urban individuals, who often face time constraints, planning meals and opting for healthy snacking options can make maintaining a balanced diet more feasible.

In conclusion, the importance of hydration and nutrition in supporting the Vagus Nerve and overall well-being cannot be overstated. A conscious approach to drinking adequate water and consuming a balanced, nutrient-rich diet can significantly enhance the nerve's function. This, in turn, can lead to better management of stress and an overall improved quality of life, especially for those in high-stress urban environments. Adopting these dietary practices offers a practical and effective way to support one's physical and mental health in the long term.

# Chapter 9: Technology and the Vagus Nerve

## Exploring modern tools for nerve stimulation

Exploring modern tools for nerve stimulation, particularly targeting the Vagus Nerve, represents a significant intersection of technology and neuroscience, offering innovative solutions for stress management and overall well-being improvement. In an age where technology pervades every aspect of life, these advancements are particularly promising for individuals in high-stress urban environments. The Vagus Nerve, an integral part of the body's parasympathetic nervous system, is crucial in managing stress responses. Stimulating this nerve can lead to decreased stress levels, improved mood, and enhanced mental health. The emergence of modern technology in this realm has introduced non-invasive, user-friendly, and accessible methods for the general public.

Among these innovations, wearable technology designed to stimulate the Vagus Nerve has gained prominence. These devices, which can be worn around the neck or on the earlobe, emit mild electrical impulses to stimulate the nerve. Designed for daily use in short sessions, they have shown promise in reducing stress, enhancing sleep quality, and improving mood.

In the realm of mobile technology, smartphone apps dedicated to relaxation and stress reduction through Vagus Nerve stimulation have become increasingly popular. These apps often combine guided breathing exercises, meditation, and biofeedback to engage the parasympathetic nervous system effectively. Additionally, the use of virtual reality (VR) is being explored to create immersive experiences that can stimulate the Vagus Nerve and induce relaxation.

Furthermore, Transcutaneous Electrical Nerve Stimulation (TENS), traditionally used for pain relief, is now being applied for Vagus Nerve stimulation. TENS devices deliver low-voltage electrical impulses through the skin, which can help reduce stress and anxiety. This approach exemplifies the innovative use of existing technology for new therapeutic applications.

The integration of technology into nerve stimulation therapies represents a significant step forward in managing stress and improving mental health. These technologies offer practical, at-home methods for engaging the Vagus Nerve, making stress management more accessible than ever. For individuals living in fast-paced urban settings, these tools provide an opportunity to integrate stress-reducing practices into their daily routines effectively.

The convergence of modern technology and nerve stimulation offers exciting possibilities for enhancing the function of the Vagus Nerve, a key player in stress response management. From wearable devices to smartphone apps and TENS units, these technologies provide innovative, practical solutions for reducing stress and promoting mental well-being. Their development and increasing accessibility are a testament to the potential of technology to positively impact health and wellness, especially in high-stress environments. As research and development in this area continue to evolve, it is likely that we will see even more advanced and effective tools for Vagus Nerve stimulation in the near future.

# Balancing technology use for mental clarity

In the contemporary era where technology is a pervasive presence in daily life, balancing its use is crucial for mental clarity and the health of the Vagus Nerve. While technology offers numerous benefits, its overuse or misuse can lead to increased stress, anxiety, and a decline in mental well-being. In the context of urban living, where the pace is fast and reliance on technology is high, it becomes essential to find a balance that fosters mental clarity and supports the health of the Vagus Nerve.

The Vagus Nerve, which plays a significant role in the parasympathetic nervous system, helps regulate stress responses and maintain a sense of calm. However, excessive exposure to digital screens, the constant connectivity, and the bombardment of information can overstimulate the nervous system, including the Vagus Nerve. This overstimulation can lead to symptoms of stress and anxiety, which in turn, can cloud mental clarity and affect overall well-being.

**Strategies for Balancing Technology Use**

To harness the benefits of technology while minimizing its stress-inducing effects, a conscious approach to its use is necessary. This involves being mindful of the time spent on digital devices and being aware of the quality of digital interactions.

**Digital Detox:** Regular intervals of digital detox, where technology use is intentionally limited, can provide the nervous system, including the Vagus Nerve, a chance to recover from digital overstimulation. This could be in the form of specific hours during the day or designated days where digital device use is minimized.

**Mindful Use of Technology:** Being mindful about technology use involves engaging with technology in a way that supports mental well-being. This includes avoiding the constant checking of emails and social media, which can lead to increased anxiety and stress.

**Quality over Quantity:** Focusing on the quality of digital interactions rather than the quantity can improve mental clarity. Engaging in meaningful digital activities that enhance learning, relaxation, and connection, rather than mindless scrolling, can positively impact mental health.

**Technology for Relaxation:** Utilizing technology for relaxation, such as apps for meditation, mindfulness, or guided breathing exercises, can actively support the health of the Vagus Nerve. These tools can provide structured ways to relax and de-stress.

**Balancing Screen Time with Physical Activity**

Balancing screen time with physical activity is another crucial aspect. Engaging in regular physical exercise, outdoor activities, or even simple walks can counteract the effects of prolonged sitting and screen exposure.

**Physical Exercise:** Regular physical activity not only improves physical health but also reduces stress and anxiety, enhancing vagal tone.

**Nature Exposure:** Spending time in nature, away from digital devices, can have a calming effect on the mind and body, supporting the function of the Vagus Nerve.

## Creating a Tech-Healthy Environment

Creating an environment that supports a healthy relationship with technology is vital. This involves setting up physical spaces where technology use is limited, such as bedrooms or certain relaxation areas in the home.

**Technology-Free Zones:** Establishing areas in the home where technology use is discouraged can create spaces for relaxation and family connection.

**Managing Notifications:** Reducing the number of notifications from apps and emails can decrease the constant sense of urgency and the need to be always connected.

In conclusion, balancing technology use is essential for maintaining mental clarity and supporting the health of the Vagus Nerve, especially for those living in high-stress urban environments. By adopting strategies such as regular digital detoxes, mindful use of technology, balancing screen time with physical activity, and creating a tech-healthy environment, individuals can enjoy the benefits of technology without compromising their mental well-being. This balanced approach is key to managing stress, enhancing vagal tone, and maintaining overall health and well-being in the modern digital age.

# Case studies: Enhancing vagus nerve health with technology

The integration of technology in enhancing the health of the Vagus Nerve, a crucial element in managing stress and promoting relaxation, has been a subject of much interest and research. Various technological advancements have been made in this field, offering innovative solutions for stimulating the Vagus Nerve and improving overall well-being. In this context, several case studies highlight the effectiveness of these technological interventions, particularly for individuals living in urban areas with high-stress lifestyles.

# Case Study 1: Wearable Tech for Stress Management

The first case involves Alex, a 40-year-old software developer from a bustling metropolitan area. Alex's job demands long hours in front of the computer, leading to chronic stress and anxiety. He started using a wearable device designed to stimulate the Vagus Nerve through mild electrical impulses. The device, which Alex wore around his neck for an hour each day, emitted gentle pulses that activated his Vagus Nerve, promoting relaxation and reducing stress levels. Over a period of six weeks, Alex reported significant improvements in his stress levels, mood, and sleep quality. He also noticed an increased ability to focus at work and a general sense of well-being.

# Case Study 2: VR for Deep Relaxation

Sarah, a 38-year-old marketing executive, faced constant deadlines and high-pressure situations at work. To manage her stress, she turned to a virtual reality (VR) program specifically designed for relaxation and Vagus Nerve stimulation. The VR experience transported Sarah to various serene environments, such as forests and beaches, where she engaged in guided relaxation and breathing exercises. The immersive nature of VR helped Sarah disconnect from her immediate stresses, allowing her to achieve a deep state of relaxation. After a month of regular use, Sarah experienced a noticeable decrease in her stress levels and an improvement in her overall mental clarity.

## Case Study 3: Smartphone Apps for Mindfulness and Breathing Exercises

John, a 45-year-old financial analyst, struggled with work-related stress and its impact on his personal life. He started using a smartphone app that offered guided mindfulness and breathing exercises aimed at stimulating the Vagus Nerve. The app's exercises, which John practiced during his lunch breaks and after work, focused on deep, diaphragmatic breathing and mindfulness techniques. These practices helped John activate his parasympathetic nervous system, reducing his anxiety and enhancing his focus. Over time, John reported feeling more in control of his stress, with improved sleep and a more positive outlook on life.

## Case Study 4: Transcutaneous Electrical Nerve Stimulation (TENS) for Relaxation

Emily, a 35-year-old teacher, experienced chronic stress, leading to physical symptoms like headaches and muscle tension. She began using a Transcutaneous Electrical Nerve Stimulation (TENS) unit, which delivered low-voltage electrical impulses to stimulate her Vagus Nerve. Emily used the TENS unit for 30 minutes each evening, focusing on areas around her neck and shoulders. The stimulation provided by the TENS unit helped alleviate her physical symptoms and induced a state of relaxation. After several weeks, Emily noticed a significant reduction in her stress-related symptoms and an improvement in her overall mood and energy levels.

These case studies illustrate the potential of technology in enhancing Vagus Nerve health and managing stress. From wearable devices and VR to smartphone apps and TENS units, technology offers various tools that can be integrated into daily routines to stimulate the Vagus Nerve and promote relaxation. For individuals in urban, high-stress environments, these technological solutions provide accessible and effective ways to manage stress, improve mental clarity, and enhance overall well-being. As technology continues to advance, it is likely that more innovative and effective solutions will emerge, further supporting the health of the Vagus Nerve and aiding in stress management.

# Part V: Your Customized Plan

# Chapter 10: Creating Your Vagus Nerve Exercise Routine

## Assessing your current mental and physical state

Assessing your current mental and physical state is a vital step in creating a Vagus Nerve exercise routine, especially for those in demanding urban environments. This process isn't just a mere evaluation; it's an essential tool that helps you understand where you stand in terms of mental and physical health and guides you in identifying the specific needs that your exercise routine should address.

Understanding the importance of this assessment is key. The Vagus Nerve, crucial in managing your body's relaxation response, is influenced by various factors, including stress levels, physical activity, diet, and overall lifestyle. Therefore, a comprehensive assessment that considers these aspects is essential in determining the appropriate exercises and interventions. For urban individuals, especially those dealing with high levels of stress, this step is crucial in tailoring a routine that effectively supports the Vagus Nerve.

The first aspect of this assessment involves evaluating your mental state. This includes understanding your stress levels, anxiety, mood patterns, and overall emotional well-being. Tools such as stress questionnaires or mood diaries can be instrumental in this process. They help in providing a clear picture of your mental health, highlighting areas that need attention. Additionally, mindfulness practices like meditation can offer insights into your mental state, helping you become more aware of your stress triggers and emotional responses.

On the physical side, assessing your current level of physical fitness, any existing health conditions, and your body's response to stress is crucial. Physical indicators such as heart rate variability, blood pressure, and even digestive health can offer clues about the state of your Vagus Nerve. In urban settings, where lifestyle can often be sedentary, this assessment helps in identifying physical limitations and areas that need strengthening or relaxation.

Lifestyle factors also play a significant role in the health of the Vagus Nerve. This includes your diet, sleep patterns, and overall daily routine. Evaluating these aspects can help you identify changes that might benefit the Vagus Nerve. For instance, incorporating a diet rich in anti-inflammatory foods, ensuring adequate sleep, and managing work-related stress are all factors that directly affect the nerve's health.

Once the assessment is complete, the information gathered can be used to tailor a Vagus Nerve exercise routine that is aligned with your specific needs. This routine might include breathing exercises, physical activities like yoga or walking, and practices aimed at reducing stress and improving mental well-being. The key is to create a balanced routine that addresses both mental and physical aspects, contributing to the overall health of the Vagus Nerve.

In conclusion, assessing your current mental and physical state is a foundational step in creating an effective Vagus Nerve exercise routine. For individuals in high-stress urban environments, this step is particularly crucial. It helps in creating a personalized routine that not only addresses current health needs but also contributes to long-term well-being. By understanding and responding to your body's and mind's unique requirements, you can effectively enhance the health of your Vagus Nerve, leading to improved stress management, better mental clarity, and overall improved quality of life.

# Tailoring exercises to your needs and goals

Tailoring exercises to meet your specific needs and goals is essential in developing an effective Vagus Nerve exercise routine, particularly crucial for those in high-stress urban environments. The Vagus Nerve, integral to the body's parasympathetic nervous system, is pivotal in stress management and emotional well-being. Crafting a personalized exercise routine requires a thorough understanding of individual mental and physical states, lifestyle, and personal objectives.

Understanding individual needs is the first step. This involves a comprehensive assessment of mental health, including stress, anxiety, or depression levels, and physical factors like fitness levels, health conditions, and overall energy. Lifestyle factors, including work environment, diet, and sleep patterns, also significantly influence the effectiveness of the exercise routine.

Setting personal goals is critical. These goals vary among individuals; some may prioritize stress reduction, others may focus on improving sleep quality or enhancing mental clarity. Clear, achievable goals guide the selection of exercises and the structure of the routine.

Several exercises effectively stimulate the Vagus Nerve. Deep, slow breathing exercises, such as diaphragmatic breathing or the 4-7-8 technique, directly stimulate the Vagus Nerve, promoting relaxation. Gentle physical exercises like yoga or tai chi not only work on the body but also on the mind, enhancing the nerve's function. Mindfulness and meditation practices help in grounding and calming the mind, further stimulating the Vagus Nerve.

For urban individuals, incorporating these exercises into a busy schedule can be challenging. Therefore, it's important to design a routine that is flexible and easily integrable into daily life. This might mean short breathing exercises during work breaks or a yoga session in the morning or evening.

The effectiveness of the routine depends on its regularity and alignment with personal needs and goals. For instance, someone dealing with high stress might benefit more from focused breathing exercises, while another individual seeking to improve digestion may find gentle physical exercises more beneficial.

Adapting the routine over time is also key. As your needs and goals evolve, so should your exercise routine. Regular reassessment of your mental and physical state can inform adjustments to the routine, ensuring it remains effective and relevant.

In conclusion, creating a personalized Vagus Nerve exercise routine is a dynamic process that requires an understanding of individual needs, setting specific goals, and choosing the right mix of exercises. For people in high-stress environments, such as urban settings, this tailored approach is particularly beneficial. It ensures that the routine not only addresses current health needs but also adapts to changing lifestyles and goals, leading to long-term improvements in stress management and overall well-being.

# Tracking progress and adapting your routine

Tracking progress and adapting your Vagus Nerve exercise routine is a critical phase in ensuring the effectiveness of your stress management strategy, especially in the context of an urban, high-stress lifestyle. This process involves regularly monitoring your mental and physical responses to the exercises, evaluating the impact on your overall well-being, and making necessary adjustments to optimize the benefits. This continuous cycle of assessment and adaptation is key to maintaining a routine that effectively supports the health of your Vagus Nerve over time.

Tracking progress in your Vagus Nerve exercise routine is crucial for several reasons. First, it helps in identifying what works best for you. Since everyone's response to stress and exercises can vary greatly, tracking allows you to understand which exercises have the most positive impact on your stress levels, mood, and overall health. Second, it keeps you motivated and committed to your routine. Seeing tangible improvements in your well-being can be a powerful motivator to continue and deepen your practice.

**Methods for Tracking Progress**

**Journaling**: Keeping a daily or weekly journal where you record your exercise routines, your feelings, stress levels, and any changes in your physical and mental state can be insightful. This record not only tracks your progress but also helps in identifying patterns and correlations between your routine and your well-being.

**Mood and Stress Questionnaires:** Using standardized questionnaires or scales to regularly rate your mood and stress levels can provide a more objective measure of your progress.

**Physical Indicators**: Monitoring physical indicators such as heart rate variability, sleep quality, and digestion can offer insights into the impact of your routine on your physical health.

**Feedback from Others:** Sometimes, changes in your well-being are noticed by those around you. Feedback from family, friends, or colleagues can provide an external perspective on any changes they observe.

## Adapting Your Routine

Adapting your Vagus Nerve exercise routine is as important as tracking your progress. As you gain insights from tracking, you might find that certain exercises are more effective than others, or that your needs and goals evolve over time.

**Adjusting Exercise Types:** Based on your tracking, you might find that certain exercises, like deep breathing, yoga, or meditation, are particularly beneficial. In such cases, you can increase their frequency or duration in your routine.

**Addressing New Goals:** As your stress levels change or as you achieve certain goals, new needs might emerge. For instance, if you initially focused on stress reduction but now want to improve sleep quality, you might incorporate specific exercises that promote better sleep.

**Experimenting with New Techniques:** The field of Vagus Nerve exercises is continuously evolving. Staying informed about new techniques and incorporating them into your routine can provide fresh perspectives and benefits.

**Seeking Professional Guidance:** If you find it challenging to adapt your routine effectively, seeking advice from professionals like therapists, yoga instructors, or wellness coaches can provide tailored guidance.

**Regular Reassessment**

Regular reassessment is crucial in this process. Set periodic check-ins, maybe every month or quarter, to review your progress and make necessary changes. During these reassessments, consider not just your immediate feelings but also long-term trends in your well-being.

In conclusion, tracking progress and adapting your Vagus Nerve exercise routine is a dynamic and ongoing process.

# Chapter 11: Integrating Practices into Daily Life

## Practical tips for busy lifestyles

Integrating Vagus Nerve exercises into a busy lifestyle can seem daunting, especially for individuals living in fast-paced urban environments. However, with practical strategies and thoughtful planning, it's entirely possible to weave these beneficial practices into your daily life, thereby enhancing mental clarity and managing stress more effectively. The key lies in finding flexible and efficient methods to include these exercises in your schedule, creating a routine that doesn't feel overwhelming or burdensome.

Starting small and focusing on consistency is crucial. Initiating your Vagus Nerve health journey with manageable exercises, even if they last only a few minutes each, can make a significant difference. Consistency is more critical than the duration of each exercise; short, daily practices are often more effective than longer, less frequent sessions.

One effective strategy is to integrate exercises into your existing daily routine. Look for moments in your day where Vagus Nerve exercises can be incorporated naturally. This could be practicing deep breathing exercises during your commute, engaging in a brief meditation session during your coffee break, or performing a quick yoga routine in the morning. The objective is to make these exercises a seamless and routine part of your day, rather than an additional task.

Technology can also be a powerful ally in maintaining your routine. Utilize smartphone apps that offer guided breathing exercises, set reminders to take short meditation breaks, or follow online yoga sessions if attending in-person classes isn't feasible. Many apps and online platforms are specifically designed to guide users through various Vagus Nerve exercises, making it easier to stay engaged and consistent.

Another practical tip is to use 'dead' time effectively. These are moments in your day that are typically unproductive, such as waiting in line, walking to the office, or even during household chores. Utilizing these moments for Vagus Nerve exercises can make your routine more efficient and less time-consuming.

Additionally, creating a supportive environment is crucial. Discuss your goals with family, friends, or colleagues who can offer support or even join you in these practices. Having a support system not only provides motivation but also helps in integrating these exercises into your social life, making them more enjoyable and sustainable.

Lastly, be adaptable and open to adjusting your routine as needed. Life in urban settings can be unpredictable, and flexibility is key to maintaining your Vagus Nerve exercise routine amidst the chaos. If you miss a session, don't be too hard on yourself. Instead, focus on getting back on track as soon as possible.

In the end, incorporating Vagus Nerve exercises into a busy urban lifestyle is about making smart, strategic choices and being consistent with your efforts. By starting small, integrating exercises into your daily routine, utilizing technology, making the most of 'dead' time, creating a supportive environment, and being adaptable, you can effectively enhance your mental clarity and manage stress, all while keeping up with the demands of your busy life.

# Building habits for long-term mental clarity

Building habits for long-term mental clarity in the fast-paced lifestyle of an urban setting can seem like a daunting task. However, with a focused approach and consistent practice, it's entirely possible to develop routines that not only enhance the health of the Vagus Nerve but also contribute significantly to mental clarity and overall well-being. This process involves understanding the principles of habit formation, implementing strategies that align with individual lifestyles, and maintaining these practices over time.

## Understanding the Science of Habit Formation

Habit formation is a process deeply rooted in psychology and neuroscience. It involves the development of behaviors that, through repetition in a consistent context, become automatic responses. The key to building lasting habits for mental clarity lies in understanding how to trigger the desired behavior (such as a Vagus Nerve exercise) and ensuring a reward or positive outcome follows it.

## Setting Realistic Goals

The first step in building these habits is setting achievable and realistic goals. These goals should be specific, measurable, attainable, relevant, and time-bound (SMART). For instance, instead of vaguely deciding to 'practice more mindfulness,' set a goal to 'perform five minutes of deep breathing exercises every morning for a month.'

## Creating a Routine

Establishing a routine is crucial. This means scheduling your Vagus Nerve exercises at the same time and place every day. Whether it's a few minutes of meditation in the morning or a brief yoga session after work, having a consistent routine helps in cementing these practices into your daily life.

## Starting Small

It's essential to start small and gradually increase the complexity and duration of the exercises. Overwhelming yourself with lengthy, complicated routines at the start can lead to frustration and abandonment of the practice. Begin with simple, short exercises that can easily be incorporated into your daily schedule.

## Cue-Routine-Reward Cycle

Understanding and utilizing the cue-routine-reward cycle is pivotal. Identify a regular cue to initiate your exercise (such as a morning alarm), follow it with your Vagus Nerve exercise routine, and then reward yourself. Rewards can be as simple as a few moments of relaxation or a healthy breakfast. This cycle helps in solidifying the habit.

## Mindfulness and Self-Compassion

Be mindful and practice self-compassion throughout this process. Building new habits is a journey that requires patience and understanding. There will be days when you might skip your routine; instead of being harsh on yourself, acknowledge the lapse and gently steer back on track.

## Leveraging Technology

In a world driven by technology, using digital tools can be highly beneficial. There are numerous apps and online platforms designed to guide and remind you about your Vagus Nerve exercises. Utilizing these tools can provide structure and consistency to your routine.

## Social Support and Accountability

Having a support system can significantly enhance your ability to stick to your routine. Share your goals with friends, family, or colleagues who can offer encouragement and hold you accountable. Sometimes, joining a group or community with similar goals can provide the necessary motivation and support.

**Regular Tracking and Adaptation**

Regularly tracking your progress is essential. Keep a journal or use an app to monitor your consistency and any changes in your mental clarity and stress levels. Be prepared to adapt your routine as needed. As your lifestyle changes, so should your exercises to ensure they remain effective and enjoyable.

**Integration into Lifestyle**

Finally, integrating these practices into your lifestyle means making them a part of your identity. Over time, as these exercises become ingrained in your daily routine, they transition from being just a habit to a part of who you are - someone who prioritizes mental well-being and clarity.

In conclusion, building habits for long-term mental clarity is a process that requires understanding the principles of habit formation, setting realistic goals, starting small, utilizing the cue-routine-reward cycle, being mindful, leveraging technology, seeking social support, regularly tracking progress, and integrating these practices into your lifestyle. With patience, consistency, and a bit of self-compassion, these practices can become a natural and rewarding part of your daily life, especially crucial in the demanding context of urban living.

# Overcoming common obstacles to consistent practice

Overcoming common obstacles to consistent practice in Vagus Nerve exercises is a crucial aspect of integrating these practices into daily life, especially for individuals in urban environments, where the pace of life can be relentless and time is a precious commodity. Consistency in practice is key to reaping the long-term benefits for mental clarity and stress reduction, but it's not uncommon to face various hurdles that can derail even the best-laid plans. Understanding these obstacles and developing strategies to overcome them is essential for maintaining a consistent routine.

## 1. Time Constraints

One of the most common obstacles is the perception of not having enough time. Urban lifestyles often involve juggling work, family responsibilities, and social commitments, leaving little room for self-care routines.

Strategy: The key is to integrate small practices into your daily routine. This could be as simple as performing a few minutes of deep breathing exercises during your commute or practicing mindfulness during a lunch break. It's about finding pockets of time and utilizing them effectively.

## 2. Lack of Motivation

There are days when motivation can be low, making it challenging to stick to your routine.

Strategy: Set small, achievable goals and celebrate when you reach them. This could be something as simple as committing to a five-minute meditation for a week and then acknowledging your accomplishment. Keeping a journal of how you feel after each practice can also serve as a motivator, as you can visually track the benefits over time.

## 3. Physical Limitations

Physical constraints, whether due to health conditions or lack of fitness, can hinder the practice of certain exercises.

Strategy: Tailor your routine to suit your physical capabilities. If certain exercises are too strenuous, modify them or focus on less physically demanding practices like guided breathing or meditation. Consulting with a healthcare provider or a fitness expert can provide insights into what exercises are most suitable for you.

## 4. Mental Barriers

Mental hurdles such as skepticism, fear of failure, or the belief that the exercises won't be effective can impede practice.

Strategy: Educate yourself about the benefits of Vagus Nerve exercises and the science behind them. Understanding how these practices impact your body and mind can help in overcoming skepticism. Start small and allow yourself to experience the benefits firsthand.

## 5. Environmental Distractions

The urban environment can be full of distractions that make it challenging to focus on relaxation exercises.

Strategy: Create a dedicated space for your practices, free from interruptions. It doesn't have to be a large space – even a small corner of a room can be transformed into a peaceful area for your exercises. Using noise-cancelling headphones or playing soft, calming music can also help in minimizing distractions.

## 6. Inconsistent Routine

An irregular routine can make it difficult to develop a habit.

Strategy: Establish a specific time each day for your exercises and stick to it. Consistency is key in habit formation. Using reminders or alarms on your phone can help in maintaining a regular schedule.

## 7. Social Expectations

Social pressures and the fear of judgment from others can sometimes prevent individuals from practicing, especially in public or shared spaces.

Strategy: Remember that your mental health and well-being are paramount. Practice in private if that's where you feel most comfortable, or find like-minded individuals or groups who share your interest in Vagus Nerve exercises. There's strength in numbers, and practicing in a group can provide additional motivation and support.

## 8. Plateauing

After some time, you might feel like your progress has plateaued, which can be discouraging.

Strategy: Mix up your routine to keep it interesting. Trying new types of exercises or increasing the intensity or duration of your practice can help in overcoming plateaus. Additionally, revisiting and possibly revising your goals can provide new motivation.

In conclusion, while there are several obstacles to maintaining a consistent practice of Vagus Nerve exercises, especially in the context of a busy urban life, these challenges can be overcome with strategic planning, motivation, and adaptability. By recognizing these common hurdles and implementing strategies to counteract them, you can ensure that your practice remains a consistent and beneficial part of your daily routine, ultimately contributing to improved mental clarity and reduced stress.

# Conclusion

As we conclude, it's vital to reflect on the journey we've embarked upon together. This book has not just been a collection of exercises and techniques; it has been a pathway to discovering the deep and profound connection between our physical well-being and our mental clarity, particularly in the context of the demanding urban lifestyles many of us lead.

The journey through these pages was designed to equip you with the knowledge and skills to stimulate your Vagus Nerve, a key element in managing stress and achieving mental clarity. But remember, the journey doesn't stop with the last page of this book. Instead, it evolves into a daily practice of integrating these techniques into your life.

Consistency in practicing the exercises outlined here is critical. The true power of these exercises is realized through regular and dedicated practice. It's about making a commitment to yourself, to prioritize your well-being amidst the chaos of city life.

Adaptation is also a crucial theme. As your life changes, so should your approach to these exercises. Whether it's due to shifts in your career, personal life, or health needs, being adaptable ensures that your routine remains relevant and effective in managing stress and enhancing mental clarity.

This book is not just a guide but a beginning, an initiation into a lifelong commitment to well-being. Taking care of your Vagus Nerve isn't a temporary fix; it's a continuous journey that requires making conscious choices every day for your health and happiness.

Sharing this knowledge with others can amplify the impact of these practices. The power of community in spreading well-being and support cannot be understated. As you experience the benefits, sharing your journey can encourage others to embark on their own paths to well-being.

In closing, remember that your path to mental clarity and stress relief is as unique as you are. Embrace the journey with its challenges and triumphs, knowing that each step you take is a move toward a more balanced and harmonious life.

Let this book serve as a foundational guide, but let your experiences and intuition lead the way. Continue to explore, adapt, and grow. Your journey to harmonizing your mind and body is one of the most rewarding endeavors, and it starts with a commitment to yourself, a single step forward into a future of clarity and calm.

www.ingramcontent.com/pod-product-compliance
Lightning Source LLC
Chambersburg PA
CBHW050729260726
48661CB00001B/135